D1076172

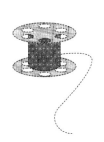

The Little Book of

SEWING

KAREN BALL

HEAD
of ZEUS

An Anima Book

This Anima book was first published in the UK
in 2019 by Head of Zeus Ltd

Copyright © Karen Ball, 2019

The moral right of Karen Ball to be identified as the author
of this work has been asserted in accordance with the
Copyright, Designs and Patents Act of 1988.

All rights reserved. No part of this publication may be
reproduced, stored in a retrieval system, or transmitted
in any form or by any means, electronic, mechanical,
photocopying, recording, or otherwise, without the prior
permission of both the copyright owner and the above
publisher of this book.

9 7 5 3 1 2 4 6 8

A catalogue record for this book is available
from the British Library.

ISBN (HB): 9781788546706
ISBN (E): 9781788546690

Designed by Lee Simmons
Ilustrations by Heather Ryerson

Printed and bound in Germany
by CPI Books GmbH

Head of Zeus Ltd
5-8 Hardwick Street
London EC1R 4RG

WWW.HEADOFZEUS.COM

To TMOS

Contents

Introduction

Acknowledgments

About the Author

INTRODUCTION

'My mom taught me to sew when I was
two or three, so I've been sewing for as
long as I can remember.'
Serena Williams

In my grandmother's house there were two instruments – a piano and a sewing machine. As a child, I sat beside her at each of these, watching her hands move across keys or beside stitches. Nana's life had been hard and she found it difficult to show love, even to little girls. But as we sat together in silence, I understood immutably that she loved me. This is the power of sewing.

When I grew older, I was allowed to sew myself – at my mother's machine, in the corner of the living room. This was the machine that made school uniforms for three daughters and outfits for dance classes. It was also the machine where I learned independent creativity for the first time.

As a student I did more sewing on a machine loaned to me by an aunt. I still sewed when I first moved to London at the age of twenty-two. Then, for some reason, I stopped. The machine was shoved into the bottom of a wardrobe, lost in a house move, and I probably didn't pick up a needle again for twenty years.

What brought me back? My career proved not to be quite enough – having it all felt kind of empty, and I needed a new creative outlet. So I found a secondhand sewing machine on Freecycle (remember Freecycle?). I picked up a heavy, clunky Toshiba with missing instructions and chipped plastic bobbins from an elderly woman in Essex. I wonder if she had any idea what she was starting, the day she handed over that machine.

Sewing has become my life. It has helped me accept my changing body, celebrate life's small joys, heal when I felt sad, mark landmark birthdays, births, weddings – and create a handmade wardrobe along the way. Sometimes, the clothes feel like an added bonus.

I have watched sewing fuel other people's passions, too. It's helped friends manage anxiety, support partners who are transgender, heal from babies born and babies lost. Sewing has empowered friends to take part on protest marches, make their voices heard, push through failure and come out the other side. It's allowed for laughter, friendship and community.

Between these pages, we'll explore the full spectrum of sewing emotions with handy practical tips thrown in – from threading a needle to fitting a dress.

And you won't only read my story of sewing. With permission, I've shared quotes from blog readers. Hopefully, you'll see how a needle and thread can change all our lives.

Sewing isn't just a hobby; it's a passion. You're about to find out just how powerful that passion can be.

Karen
of *Did You Make That*

CHAPTER 1

ASPIRATION

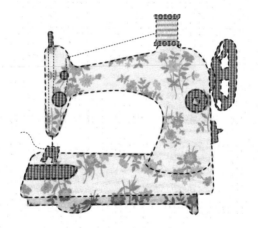

To aspire is one of the greatest gifts we can give ourselves. It gives us purpose, hope, inspiration and a plan for self-improvement. Aspiration puts the hunger in our belly and allows us to dream big. But it doesn't need to start big – baby steps are fine right now. You learn how to thread a needle or tie a knot. That's how it begins. Before you know it, you're sewing a couture evening gown. Be brave in your aspirations, because this is only the start of the journey. It's going to take you places you hardly dared dream of...

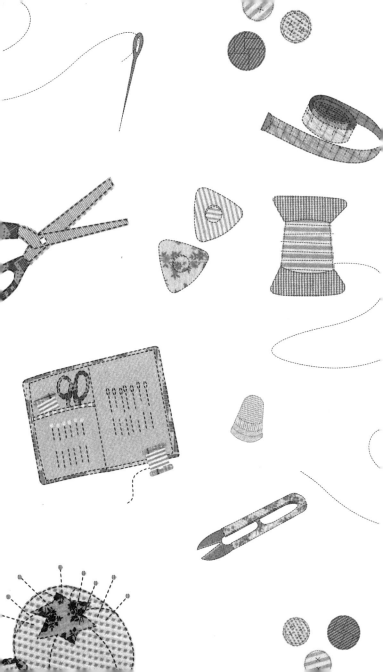

Can anyone sew?

How to choose thread

What is a sewing pattern?

How to thread a needle

Your first needle case

Setting goals

How to knot a thread

New and fearless

Tips for improvement

You will learn:

How to choose thread
How to thread a needle
How to knot a thread

CAN ANYONE SEW?

'It's sort of comical that you think you made a choice that exempts you from the fashion industry, when in fact you're wearing a sweater that was chosen for you by the people in this room.'
Miranda Priestly, The Devil Wears Prada

For most of your existence up to this point, the high street has curated your clothes. Now, you've decided to do that work alone. When you're stood in the foothills, that mountain peak can look exhilarating. It can also look scary. You ask yourself: 'Can I really do this? Can anyone sew?'

Yes, anyone can sew. YOU can sew. Don't let fear of failure stop you. Just remember...

Baby steps

'The most difficult thing is the decision to act. The rest is merely tenacity.'
Amelia Earhart, female explorer

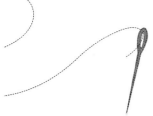

Take it one step at a time. Did Amelia Earhart become the first woman to fly across the Atlantic by looking at a two-seater biplane and whimpering, 'But I don't know where the brakes are?'

Failure is necessary

No one learned anything by being perfect. You will fail. You will curse. You will bunch your fabric up and hurl it into a corner of the room. Then you'll calm down, dust yourself off and try again.

'Enjoy failure and learn from it. You can never learn from success.' James Dyson

The joy is in the doing

It doesn't matter if your first sewing project isn't perfect. You made something with your very own hands. Yes, YOU. The world disappeared and for a few precious hours, the only thing that filled your heart, mind and soul was sewing. How did that make you feel? Happy?

If sewing makes you happy, that means you can sew. That's all you need to know.

HOW TO CHOOSE THREAD

Ever wondered what your clothes are sewn together with? Until I began sewing, I never gave it a thought. I mean, seriously, why would you? Thread is one of those details you never consider until you have to.

But the first time you walk into a haberdashery shop, the choices seem overwhelming. Cotton? Polyester? Elastic? Decorative? Topstitching? Upholstery? Clear? And what's even with those giant cones of overlocker thread? I had to phone my mum from the shop for help. Awk.

So what should you choose?

Types of thread

All-purpose: Does what it says on the can. Typically, this is a cotton thread with a polyester coating. The polyester gives the thread a sheen that helps it travel through fabric more easily and makes the cotton longer lasting.

Polyester: Strong, durable and with a slight amount of give that helps your thread mould to the shape of a seam. Be careful with the heat of your iron – polyester can melt.

Cotton: If you believe that your thread should match your fabric type, you'll want to use cotton thread with an all-cotton project, such as a quilt. Beware, though – cheap cotton thread can be coarse, hairy and snap easily.

Silk: A pricier option, but don't mistake investment for luxury – I always have a few spools of silk thread in the house. Silk is great for any hand stitching or tacking pieces together. (Tacking refers to temporary stitches, sewn with a long stitch length by hand or on a machine.) The silk thread's high sheen makes it extra slippery and therefore easy to remove. This also means that it rarely leaves behind puncture marks in your fabric.

Topstitching: At some point in your sewing career, you'll want to do some fancy topstitching. It's so much fun! Proper topstitching thread makes a real difference – it's thicker and makes more of a visual impact.

Overlocking: Overlockers (or sergers) use multiple large cones of extra-fine thread. Don't be tempted to use sewing machine spools of thread on your overlocker, as the thread will be too thick.

Favourite thread: My favourites are high-quality polyester threads from the German company, Gutermann.

Matching thread to fabric

When choosing thread, pull out a strand from the spool and lay it across the fabric. A single strand gives a much better indication of colour matching than holding the entire spool against the fabric.

If you have to choose between two colourways

(for example, if you had to choose thread for a grey and lemon print fabric), a good rule of thumb is to go with the lighter colour of thread.

Threads on show

Your collection of spools will quickly grow. To keep your thread neatly organized (and make for a pretty display), you could consider a wooden thread rack where each spool is arranged on its own spindle. Just make sure you have a dust cover.

A final word on threads

As with many things in life, you get what you pay for. Those cheap spools on the market will give you linty threads that snap and catch in your machine. If I ever have problems with how my machine is sewing, the first check I do is the thread – switching up to a better quality thread often solves the issue.

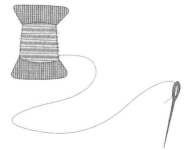

WHAT IS A SEWING PATTERN?

There are two main choices available to sewists today: a downloadable PDF to print out at home or in a copy shop, and a paper pattern. Typically, they come with a set of instructions and paper pieces that you pin out or weigh down onto fabric and cut around. This is your template for sewing an item of clothing.

As well as the Big Four pattern companies – McCalls, Vogue, Simplicity and Butterick – there has been an explosion in Indie sewing pattern companies, each offering different options of aesthetic and engagement. There has never been a better time to sew – but how do you choose your first project?

Look inside your wardrobe

What do you already like wearing? Take a look at the items that suit you and your lifestyle and choose an outfit that you know will give you lots of pleasure. Then narrow down your pattern choices accordingly.

Take inspiration from fabric

The world of sewing can be neatly divided into two tribes – those who start with a pattern and then choose fabric, and those who buy fabric and then twin it with a pattern. If you find that you're drowning in pattern options, consider a spontaneous splurge on two metres of something that makes your heart skip.

See beyond the pattern sketches

Some sewing patterns come with beautiful sketches on the envelope; some come with heinously dated styling. Both present their challenges. Beware the 1940s vintage sewing pattern featuring the model with the waspish waist – how often do you wear corsets in your daily life? Equally, try to see past a badly styled and dated photograph. Instead, turn the envelope over and inspect the pattern's line drawing. Can you see the potential? This is where a good imagination comes in useful!

Read online reviews

The Internet is your friend here. Google a pattern and see what other people have made. Do you feel inspired? There's no shame in copying - imitation is the best form of flattery. It's also a really great way of exploring your creativity until you find the confidence to pursue your own sense of style. Most authors start out by imitating a writer they admire; the same can be true of sewing.

HOW TO THREAD A NEEDLE

You don't need a sewing machine to begin sewing. You can sit on the sofa with a needle and thread.

Length of thread

Hold the spool against the tip of your chin and unravel a length of thread that reaches out as far as an outstretched arm. (Imagine yourself doing Usain Bolt's lightning pose.) If your cut thread is any longer than this, it will become unwieldy.

Divide the work

When hand stitching a detail like a hem, it's a good idea to divide your work into two or three sections of thread. If you attempt to work with one huge length of thread, it will just knot. Plus, with this technique you are future proofing your hard work: if one part of the stitching ever comes undone, you can be confident that your whole hem won't unravel.

Thread heaven

This is a wax product that stops your thread from knotting. Buy some. Run your thread through it. Avoid knots. Sometimes, life really is that easy.

Good light

Ideally daylight, but in the winter a decent daylight lamp may just save your sanity. The most dedicated sewists swear by a head torch!

Snipping

Cut your thread with sharp scissors or snippers at a 45-degree angle. The angled cut gives your thread a fine point. Grasp your thread close to the end and moisten the tip. Then, angle your needle so that you can clearly see the eye – a pale fabric or surface behind your work will help. Pass the end of your thread through the eye of your needle.

Congratulations! You've just threaded a needle.

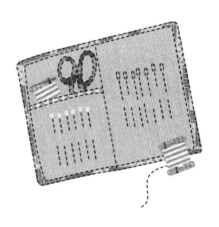

YOUR FIRST NEEDLE CASE

Do you remember your first needle case? Was it gifted to you as a child, borrowed from your mother or inherited from a grandparent? Maybe your first needle case is the one you buy as an adult, when you decide that sitting at a computer for eight-hour stretches is no longer good for your soul.

I picked out my first felt needle case on the third floor of Liberty of London. It was the only item in the store I could afford, emblematic of this new venture in my life. Now it's a chewed-up thing, mangled back when my dog was a puppy. (Yes, my dog chewed needles. Yes, I'm a bad dog owner.)

Between the felt pages of the needle case is my collection of needles. Embroidery needles, slender as a whisper and bent concave by the pressure of my hands from hand stitching countless hems. Tapestry needles, which I never make tapestries with – their blunt points are useful for threading elastic down tunnels of fabric like waistbands.

Tiny Japanese needles, their glinting eyes dipped in gold, which I use for... actually, I rarely use them for anything. They're too tiny!

You'll enjoy curating your collection of hand sewing needles more than you can imagine. They become old friends you can't bear to get rid of. You'll have a favourite, even though you claim to love them all equally. And that ratty needle case becomes as important in your household as the manual for the dishwasher - the only difference being that you always know where your needle case is.

My top hand sewing needles

'If something exists, somebody somewhere collects them.'

Unknown

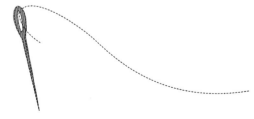

Needles come in different sizes. The bigger the number, the finer the needle. Once you start investing in your needle collection, you'll realize just how many needles there are in the world – and you'll probably want to own one of each.

A pack of assorted craft needles is all a beginner – or an experienced sewist – needs. But where's the fun in that?

I love an embroidery needle for creating tiny hand stitches that melt away into the fabric. An embroidery needle also has a long eye, which makes it easier to thread.

Hotel sewing-kit needles – a good first source of general-use needles, though the needles may rust over time.

Gold-plated needles – the gold plate allows the needle to slip easily through fabric.

Tulip needles – tiny, sharp, Japanese needles made of nickel-plated steel. They come in a tiny corked glass tube. Drop one of these at your peril, because you'll struggle to find it again.

Yes, it's easy to ritualize hand-stitching needles. What's wrong with that?

SETTING GOALS

Aspiration is nothing without goals. Goals give you direction and focus. Your goal is the HOW of sewing and your aspiration is the WHY.

Why do you aspire to sew? Is it to enjoy the satisfaction of making something with your own hands? Do you have a social conscience around fast fashion or ethical sourcing of materials? Is this your way of showing love to a new partner, baby or home? Do you need a meditative activity? Or do you want to make clothes that you can't find on the high street? Probably, it's a combination of factors – but understanding your aspirations can help you set your goals.

Write down your aspirations

Now, you can choose your goals. Your goals might be to take a class, sew an outfit, work with a challenging fabric, learn a new skill...

Write down your goals

Writing things down makes you accountable and gives you a chance to evaluate. Do those goals make your heart sing with joy or sink in your chest? Don't overthink this and don't judge yourself by other people's standards. If your goal is to sew a fancy-dress costume for your dog, you're already winning at life. Who else do you know who sews a fancy-dress costume for their dog?

Choose a sewing goal and set out to achieve it.

HOW TO KNOT A THREAD

I once spent time with a dressmaker in California who'd been sewing for over forty years. She dedicated several days to helping me sew a vintage

1960s dress suit. Our first lesson? How to knot a thread.

I've been using her technique ever since, and now I can share it with you.

- Thread your needle.

- Bring the tail of the thread around to the back of your needle and keep it there with the pad of your finger.

- With your free hand, grasp the thread. Twist it twice around the needle above the tail of thread, which is still kept pressed against the needle.

- Pull the twists of thread down the needle, off the needle and down the length of thread. This action will drag the tail of the thread along, too, until your thread pulls taut and you have... a knot at the end!

- It's that quick. That simple. You'll never have to squint or curse again.

NEW AND FEARLESS

Do you remember the first time you fell in love? With your body and soul, no fear of heartbreak? First love only happens once – and it can be the same with sewing.

I miss those new and fearless days. I miss the confidence and vigour with which I threw myself into my first sewing projects. The dress with the wonky hem and badly inserted zip: I wore it, striding down a sunny London street, and I felt awesome. A friend of mine sewed a wedding dress for her best friend as her first sewing project. A. Wedding. Dress. For. Her. Best. Friend. And you know what? She pulled it off. Would she do the same again, knowing what she knows now?

When you dig deeper into sewing, you practise your skill and improve. But the danger is that you also become more aware of the potential mistakes. You get cautious and stop taking risks.

So, I'm here to tell you – stay new and fearless. Here's how.

Don't worry about waste

Controversial, in this era of recycling, but bear with me. One of the reasons we become cautious is that we worry about wasting fabric, wasting time, wasting our creativity. But there is no waste when it comes to learning. There is no wasted time at the sewing machine. See page 216 for suggestions of what you can do with makes you won't wear.

Ignore your inner critic

Sewing brings out your inner perfectionist. I can promise you now, you'll never sew the perfect item. I haven't! It's easy to get to the end of a project and see all your mistakes, but after a few wears you'll love your handmade clothes and forget the details that didn't work. (Most of the time!)

Don't apologize

This is a particularly female trait and one I'd love to see us banish. I have read far too many sewing blog posts that open with an apology. What are you apologizing for? You created a 3-D object from scratch on your own. I call that a success!

Remember – be fearless.

TIPS FOR IMPROVEMENT

Of course, there are many simple tips and tricks for improving your sewing. If you turn these techniques into habits, they quickly become muscle memory that make all your sewing projects look 100 per cent better without you even having to think about it.

Cut accurately

A good pair of scissors can be your friend for life. Alternatively, invest in a rotary cutter and cutting mat. But whichever option you choose, accuracy makes all the difference. I began my sewing career cutting out on my living-room floor – back breaking and messy. So if you can find a table to work on, your sewing will also ascend to new heights.

Pay attention

A good set of pattern instructions will tell you what the seam allowance is – follow it! For my first sewing project, I didn't even know what a seam allowance was. Typically, it's 15 millimetres (5/8 in.), but some patterns use a smaller or larger seam allowance, so always read the instructions first. This can make or break fit.

Grade seams

This is such a deal breaker for me. When pattern instructions tell you to trim or grade seams, don't skip this step. It gets rid of a lot of unnecessary bulk that can make a real difference to the way that a seam or hem sits. I always marvel at how much fabric I throw away whenever I trim a seam. Why do you want all that extra *stuff* needlessly sitting around your body?

Press your seams

There's not a seam in the world that didn't look better for coming into contact with a hot iron. Press each seam as it's sewn – don't wait to press the finished article. But make sure that the heat of your iron matches the fibre content of your fabric. Scorched fabric never looks cool! (You can see more pressing tips on page 213.)

Don't rush

Take your time. Sew when your brain is fresh. And don't skip tacking – a technique using long stitches that allows you to judge the fit and placement of pattern pieces. If things aren't working, it's easy to rip the tacking stitches out.

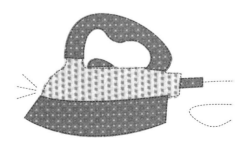

CHAPTER 2

SELF-LOVE

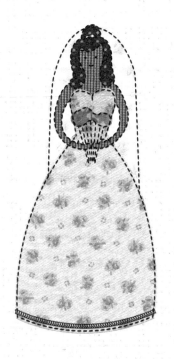

Organizing your working space is the best way to propel yourself into sewing your dream wardrobe. You may not have a dedicated room or even a table, but by gathering your arsenal you make an important statement of intent.

I can and shall sew!

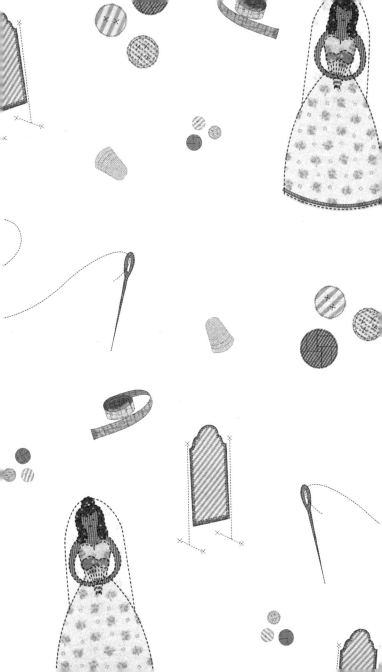

How to choose a sewing machine

Embracing creativity

Dealing with anxiety

Essential sewing tools

Juggling sewing and life

A space of your own

Podcasts to pin to

Confident sewing

Storing sewing patterns

You will learn:

How to choose a sewing machine
Your essential sewing tools
How to organize your sewing room
Tips for storing patterns

HOW TO CHOOSE A
SEWING MACHINE

'A sewing machine is essential to
every woman who is keen on sewing.'
Remy Nicholson, *A Textbook Of Dressmaking*, 1936

Do sewing machines have personalities? There's the vintage workhorse, the computerized whizz kid, the inherited keepsake, the basic essential that never lets you down. Yes, your sewing machine is your friend. And, like choosing friends, picking a sewing machine can feel like one of the biggest decisions you'll make. Here are a few tips...

Try on for size

Most serious sewists have a second (or even third or fourth!) machine stashed away in the understairs cupboard. Other friends may own an inherited machine or one they don't use any more. Put a call out amongst friends and family and see who'd be willing to loan you a machine before you buy one.

Source a freebie

You can find free sewing machines via swapping websites – that's what I did! Write an ad and see what comes back. As long as you have transport (remember, sewing machines can be heavy), this could be your quickest route to a free machine that you don't have to give back.

Sewing schools

Remember your first day at a new school, gazing around the playground and wondering who would become your best friend? One of the great things about learning to sew is that you get to experience that back-to-school vibe all over again! And attending a class at a sewing school allows you to try out their machines. This can be a great shortcut to understanding what a machine feels like to use and what you're looking for. Most schools have basic but hardworking models that could also be perfect for your needs.

Sewing machine specialists

Believe it or not, there are still high-street repair shops where you'll find expert staff who have been dealing with sewing machines for decades. Pay them a visit and benefit from their insights and wisdom. To find out about these shops, put a call out on social media for personal recommendations.

Stay in budget

You don't need to splurge thousands of pounds on your first sewing machine. Some of the best sewists I know still work on inherited models that are decades old. Others swear by their computerized gizmos. Choose your budget and stick to it.

Does brand matter?

Brands denote reliability, recommendation and reputation – at least in the world of sewing machines. Branded machines also mean that when you purchase, you're giving yourself access to after-sales support from specialists and the brand themselves. So do some research and decide which brand is for you.

> 'My mom's 1908 treadle machine still works just fine and does a beautiful straight stitch. It was bought for her second hand by my father when they got married in 1946. I learned to sew on it as a child, and made most of my clothes as a teenager using it. Eventually I inherited it, had the woodwork refurbished, and gave it pride of place in my living room.'
>
> Blog reader, Cherry

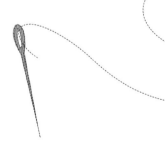

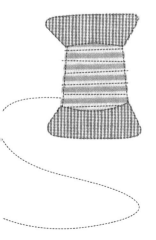

EMBRACING CREATIVITY

*'Take a risk, dare to fail and
give it your all.'*
Matthew Syed, *You Are Awesome*, 2018

You can have all the equipment in the world, but then there's the fear. No one tells you about that. It can be the biggest obstacle to fully embracing your creativity. Do any of these scenarios sound familiar to you?

- I'm worried about wasting fabric

- What if it doesn't fit?

- Will people laugh at me?

- I might make mistakes

Let me save you a bit of worrying time. You will waste fabric. You MIGHT make a dress that doesn't fit properly – that's how you learn about fit. If people laugh at you, are they really your friends? You WILL make mistakes. This is all good.

Fear of failure is the biggest obstacle to engaging with your creativity. Move that obstacle out of the way. Go ahead, fail. Life isn't an Instagram photo – it's a big, gnarly mess and sometimes your sewing will be the same.

You might feel anxious about picking up a needle, but I promise that once you let go of the fear, ridding yourself of anxiety is just one of the many benefits of sewing. Let me explain...

DEALING WITH ANXIETY

You can't sew if you're anxious; you can't be anxious if you sew.

In 2013 there were 8.2 million cases of anxiety in the UK, but being mindful is proven to reduce anxiety. What does being mindful mean? It means devoting time to your thoughts and feelings, often by engaging in a deliberate activity that you pay attention to without judging. Sound like sewing?

From personal experience, I know that sewing can be a brilliant way of dealing with anxiety.

When world or life events beyond my control agitate me, I take out a piece of sewing. Often, I turn to a smaller task that forces me to work slowly and concentrate but isn't as mentally taxing as, say, trying to ease in a sleeve head or neatly insert a zip.

Examples of mindful sewing tasks might be:

- Hand stitching a hem

- Cutting out pattern pieces

- Tacking temporary stitches

- Embroidering a motif

If you want your sewing space to be your sanctuary, build slow sewing into your acts of self-love. Your serotonin levels will thank you!

> 'I am always aware that I am continuing a tradition that human beings have learned all over the world for centuries. What we are doing is both important and inconsequential.'
> Blog reader, Rachel Begley

ESSENTIAL SEWING TOOLS

'As large a table as possible, a pair of sharp scissors, medium or large size, a piece of tailor's chalk, and a good supply of fine pins – these are the four essential things...'
Remy Nicholson, *A Textbook Of Dressmaking*, 1936

All the gear and no idea? You don't have to be that person with sewing. You don't have to buy straight away, though. Most of us have friends who can advise, recommend and loan. You'll be amazed at how much sewing wisdom and hand-me-down tools are lurking behind closed doors.

Pinking scissors

These are scissors with a saw-toothed blade that leave a zig-zag edge on any seam you cut. This edge helps to stop fabric from fraying, and allows you to finish seams even if you don't have an overlocker (serger). It's one of my favourite fun activities to spot the pinked seams in vintage handmade dresses!

Pins and pincushion

One of my oldest sewing friends swears by freshly sharp pins. The moment a pin resists puncturing fabric, she tosses it – thanks to advice from her seamstress mother. I advise the same! Don't take your pins for granted. Glass-headed pins are good if you want to avoid melting your pin heads when they inadvertently come in touch with an iron. My personal favourites are silk pins – so fine and slender, you won't want to drop one.

Your pincushions? I owned ten, last time I counted...

Measuring tape

This is something to buy new! Old tapes were often made of waxed cloth and stretch and distort over time. You want your body measurements to be accurate if you're going to accurately fit makes.

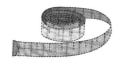

Iron and ironing board

You don't need more than the basics, but make sure your iron is clean and only using filtered water if you live in a hard-water area. I've had too many irons spit residue onto cherished makes!

Marking tools

It's easy to disappear down a rabbit warren of marking tools – chalk, chalk pens, tracing wheel and carbon paper, silk thread for tacking – but here's my top tip. Visit your local stationery shop or supermarket and buy some Frixion pens. They last a lifetime, but their marks don't – they disappear like magic beneath the heat of an iron!

That's it. You're good to go. If you have all of these, you can sew a dress. And it's my guess that most of these you already have in the house. So, honestly, the only thing you need to invest in is a pair of pinking scissors. I borrowed my first pair from my mum. In fact, I still have them!

JUGGLING SEWING AND LIFE

You have all the essential equipment, you've sourced a sewing machine and found a corner of the home to call your own. Great - now you can start sewing the outfits you've always dreamed of! Right?

Then your pet gets sick, you have to put in some overtime, your partner is asking why they don't see enough of you and the train home gets delayed. By the time you've eaten dinner and hit your sofa, you just about have enough energy to pick up the remote and change channels. Pick up a needle? You have to be kidding.

Yup, there's that little thing called life and it has a habit of getting in the way of sewing. Sometimes, for good reason: when it's a beautiful summer day, I'm ordering you to step away from the sewing machine! Sometimes you can't find time to sew for more challenging reasons.

But by this stage you've probably worked out that sewing is good for you - for your health, sanity and sense of self. Without sewing, you don't even know who you are any more! (Yup. It creeps up on you like that. Hey, there are worse addictions...)

The 15-minute rule

An oldie, but a goodie. Carve out 15 minutes a day to complete a sewing task. Pin a seam. Change the thread in your sewing machine. Apply some interfacing. You'd be amazed how these small tasks stack up and keep you feeling connected with an activity that makes you happy.

Just say no

Turn down the invitation that you don't really fancy. Politely decline the request to help out at an event. Remind your kids that they're old enough to make their own breakfast. There are lots of reasons you can say no and commit to the only thing you actually want to do - sew! Don't turn the 'no' into a conversation and don't apologize. Make your no quick, simple and polite. Then say yes to sewing.

Recognize your best and worst times

Are you a morning person or a night owl? When does your brain work best? I love to get up early and sew before the rest of the world is awake; I can't sew past 9 p.m. without making mistakes. Recognizing my own body clock and energy patterns helps make the most of the time when I can sew. If you had to choose a time in the day to sew, when would it be? Then carve out that time.

Sew together

A shared sewing activity can force you and the people around you to accommodate a pastime that makes you happy. It's a bit like a book club, exercise class or dog walking. No one would tell you not to do those, so why not make the same ring fence around your sewing time – by meeting up with friends and sewing together?

Don't beat yourself up

Hey, sometimes life is just too crazy for you to sew. Don't beat yourself up about it. You started this as a hobby, not a task. That sewing machine isn't going anywhere. It will still be there, waiting for you, when you're ready.

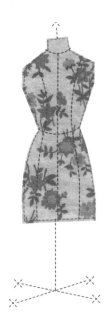

A SPACE OF YOUR OWN

Do you have a dedicated sewing room? A corner of the living room? A kitchen table that needs clearing of sewing detritus in time for every family meal? You might live in a flat share, a city apartment, a farmhouse, a condo... Some people drag their sewing machine outside, some of us sew in the basement. I've even seen people take their sewing machine on holiday.

The first rule of sewing spaces is that there are no rules of sewing spaces. But I'd recommend that you aim to make it an inspiring, clutter-free place to be. I'm not just talking vintage sewing pattern covers to decorate the walls or pretty cushions for your chairs. What are the practical steps you can take to make your sewing space a properly functioning environment?

Ergonomic Chair: The great thing about sewing is that it takes you away from the computer screen – but you're still going to do a lot of time bent over a table. First things first: make sure that your table and machine are set at the right height. Also, that it's easy to adjust your chair. You don't have to spend a fortune on an ergonomic chair, but you should invest in one. Your back and shoulders will thank you for it.

Cutting Table: If you have a waist-height cutting-out table, you are truly living the dream. Few of us have the space for this type of luxury. You can cut out kneeling on the floor, but that is back breaking indeed. My suggestion is to get a decent-sized table and a cutting mat – somewhere you can lay fabric flat for accurate pinning and cutting out. You might even consider a collapsible painter and decorator's trestle table.

Daylight Bulbs: During the winter months, you'll discover just how hard on the eyes sewing can be – especially if you're sewing with dark colours. A flexible lamp with a daylight bulb might just become your new best friend. Any lamp with a bulb you can angle will prove useful. I have four or five lamps in my living room, for just this reason.

Storage Solutions: A certain Swedish furniture company is about to become your new best friend! The holy grail of sewing is good storage. Vintage patterns need protecting from sunlight, threads need saving from becoming a bird's nest of knots, buttons, zips, interfacing, pins, PDF print-outs... All of these items need careful storage. Jars, drawers, wheeled trays, wall-mounted shelves, butchers' hooks... Get ready with your screwdriver – you'll fast improve your assembly skills once you start sewing. And we haven't even touched on fabric storage!

Don't Look Over The Garden Fence

It's easy to suffer from FOMO (Fear Of Missing Out) when you see other people's sewing spaces on social media. Do remember that we all lead different lives in different spaces and that most work environments don't stay tidy for long. Live your best life in the space you have – and be proud of what you achieve there.

'When my sewing space is chaotic, my mind feels the same way and I don't work as well. I dream of the day I can sew in my own office or studio. One day, one day...'

Blog reader, DavyMade

PODCASTS TO PIN TO

The great thing about sewing is that you don't have to work in silence – you have just enough head space to enjoy music or podcasts as you work on your latest project. Here's my run down of the best podcasts to sew to.

A Stitcher's Brew

www.stitchersbrewpodcast.co.uk/

Double acts make for brilliant podcasts, and Gabby and Megan prove that they can double that rule! As well as co-hosting as a pair, they often feature guests two at a time in this fun, informative and original sewing podcast. Between the laughs, there is lots of rich content – and added fun from Gabby's dog, Hobbes.

Love To Sew

www.lovetosewpodcast.com/

A weekly podcast hosted by Helen and Caroline, who chat with interviewees about making clothes, the online community and small businesses. Between them they also run a fabric store, host a blog and design sewing patterns.

While She Naps

www.whileshenaps.com/category/the-podcast/episodes

The host, Abby Glassenberg, takes her journalism seriously and this is reflected in her podcast, in which she doesn't shy away from the difficult questions. Always polite, always professional, she looks at the business of sewing as much as the craft.

Blogtacular

www.blogtacular.com/podcast/

The Blogtacular platform engages with creators working online. If you ever wanted to know how creatives manage their careers, what impact social media has and how to engage with an online community, this podcast allows you to peek behind the curtain of the craft industry. Plus, it's fun!

In Good Company

www.womenwho.co/podcast/

Otegha Uwagba is the author of *Little Black Book, A Toolkit For Working Women* and she brings a ferociously intelligent eye to women's careers. Relevant to any woman who is considering her place in life and work, Otegha shares advice that is both insightful and compassionate.

The High Low

www.dollyalderton.com

Dolly Alderton teams up with her pal, Pandora Sykes, in this weekly podcast that covers a range of news items that have caught their eye. They are intelligent and witty and their friendship allows the podcast to feel intimate and edgy – you never quite know what one of them will say next.

How To Fail Podcast

www.howtofail.podbean.com

Elizabeth Day interviews celebrated creatives about key events in their lives when they failed, and how that influenced them - a fascinating and humbling listen.

CONFIDENT SEWING

'Awesome is a choice we make.'
Blog reader, Kathryn Gutteridge

Sewing impacts on your self-love in all sorts of ways. The outfits you might have dismissed in a previous life suddenly become your favourite new makes. You begin to question style rules and fashion proclamations about what you should wear and when. The only person curating your wardrobe is you - and it's no coincidence that your confidence goes through the roof!

Body measurements

You become more intimate with your body measurements than you ever have been at any other point in your life – not because you want to judge yourself by these numbers, but because they're your tool for success. Sewing is a brilliant way of stripping judgement out of the tape measure.

You made that

You can step out of the house wearing something that you made with your own two hands. No one else in the world has one of what you just created – a 3-D object from fabric. What does that say about you? That you're awesome. No one can deny that – not even your inner voice.

Aspire, then achieve

One of the first things I noticed about sewing is that it allowed me to aspire to greatness I never had to consider was beyond me. I saw other people's makes on the Internet and my mind was blown. These were normal people making incredible outfits. If those normal people could be incredible ... maybe I could, too.

Watch yourself improve

A great reason to set up a blog or social media profile is that you have a visual diary of your sewing journey. You will see yourself improve and enjoy being cheered on by others. With application, practice and energy, you can only go one way. It's often difficult to track meaningful progress in other parts of your life, especially when so many jobs exist only on a computer – but the more you sew, the more you see yourself improve. When was the last time you were able to award yourself a gold star?

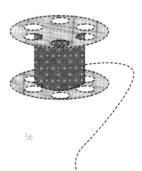

STORING SEWING PATTERNS

I'm not going to lie – once you buy your first sewing pattern, you're opening Pandora's box. You'll find yourself scouring secondhand auction websites for rare vintage finds, clicking the Order button for downloadable PDFs, taking advantage of pattern sales and generally stockpiling a whole selection of cardboard envelopes with pretty line drawings.

Before you know it, you'll have towering piles of patterns spilling all over your home. But if you're going to invest, you need to take care of your burgeoning collection.

Vintage patterns

Store these out of daylight and in acid-free protective bags, either in hanging files or cardboard boxes. If you're anxious to preserve the pattern pieces, trace them off before you use them. You might even want to photocopy the instructions to make sure that the original doesn't get damaged with use. Old, yellowing paper crumbles easily.

Top tip: Look out for old pins, notes or even love letters amongst your vintage sewing patterns!

PDF print-outs

These can be ultra bulky. I roll mine up and keep them stored in a sideboard. Alternatively, pattern hooks and hangers can keep the large pattern pieces stored out of your way.

Pattern Companies

The Big Four refers to the largest pattern companies – McCalls, Vogue, Simplicity and Butterick. Indie pattern companies are single-person or small-team start-ups, designing and producing their own spin on sewing patterns. Most of these companies produce paper patterns that come in A3 envelopes or slip cases. Some can be beautiful, others less so! All of them need to be stored somewhere safe.

Look out for attractive storage boxes in the sales and stack them up. Some people file their patterns and keep a catalogue. I just try to make sure that my patterns are in easy reach to flip through when I'm looking for inspiration.

Try to keep tidy

It's tricky, I know, but try to keep on top of your storage. The people you live with will thank you and you'll avoid loss, damage or simply forgetting what you already own. Yes, I know people who have multiple copies of sewing patterns – simply because they can't remember what they've already bought. Don't let this be you!

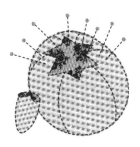

CHAPTER 3

BODY IMAGE

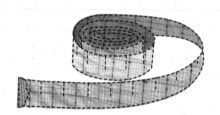

Learning how to sew means learning how to
love your body. When you're no longer obliged
to rely on variable high-street clothes sizing,
you can sew to suit the body you were born
with or the body you've created.
Okay, guys and gals and everyone
in between – prepare to have
your mind exploded!

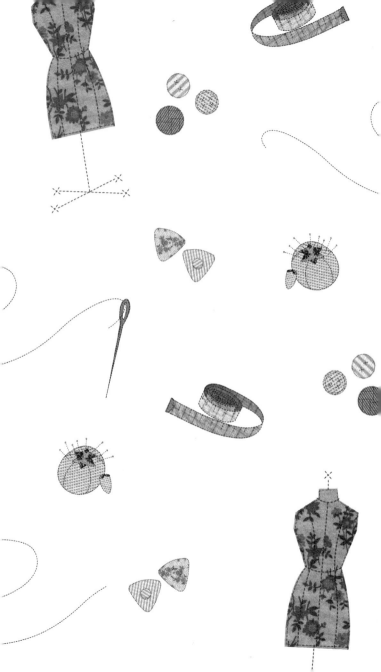

Your body as a toolbox

Naked sewing

The best body measuring tools

Choosing a pattern size

Food and sewing

Fitting techniques

Every body's wonky

Sexuality and sewing

Three common fitting adjustments

Your changing body

You will learn:

How to take accurate body measurements

Tissue fitting

How to sew a toile

Common fitting adjustments

YOUR BODY AS A TOOLBOX

Forget investing in a state-of-the-art sewing machine. When it comes to sewing and a positive self-image, your greatest toolbox is your body – that strong, powerful miracle of nature that steers you through life, day after day and year after year.

If you've ever judged your body by its failings – too tall, too short, too fat, too thin, too broken – sewing is about to turn all your preconceptions on their head and send your confidence through the roof.

When you start sewing, you'll need to take accurate body measurements. For the first time in years, you'll know rather than guess what your chest, waist and hip measurements are.

You'll look in the mirror and be able to see how your body is totally unique – the wonky shoulder from a childhood fall, the scar from an operation, the mummy tummy. These aren't failings – these are sewing opportunities. Over time, your body becomes an engineering challenge rather than an exercise in failure. And once you understand how to sew the most flattering outfits for you, there's no looking back.

Your body is a toolbox. Are you ready to open the lid to happiness?

NAKED SEWING

'A hot evening at one of my pattern cutting classes, six students including one very pregnant lady sat in their underwear making toiles...'
Sewing Teacher, Alice

If you're going to sew, you'll need to get naked – a lot! Any sewing project usually means trying on your work in progress for fit, and if you are sewing in a group, you may be getting changed in company. I've changed in toilets, offices and even in front windows!

So you'd better get used to seeing bare flesh – yours and other people's. Hey, we're all friends.

Here's how to handle your jiggly bits with decorum - or not.

Mirrors

You can never have too many mirrors in a sewing household and, if you're clever, you can position them in a place that guarantees you maximum privacy. I know exactly the spot in my living room where I can peel off my clothes without scaring the neighbours. Get tactical with the layout of your sewing space.

Make it easy on yourself

If you are going to be climbing in and out of day wear, maybe think about what outfit you choose in the morning. A simple T-shirt dress that can be whipped over your head is ideal. A complicated outfit that involves buttons, buckles and layers? Not so great.

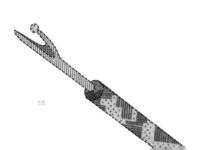

Draw the curtains

When you're fitting a project, you're peeling off and putting on layers again and again – and again! You may decide there's no point climbing back into your day clothes. You may decide it's easiest to sew in your underwear. We've all done it.

Just make sure you draw the curtains and warn family members before they enter the sewing space. Or maybe you just don't care. My sewing machine sits beside a window. I've sewn in my bra and knickers before now, daring a neighbour to glance through the window. Hey – if they choose to look, they're going to have to face the consequences.

Underwear

Remember what your mum used to tell you about wearing clean underwear? If you got knocked over, you wouldn't want the ambulance man to see you in less than your best knickers. It's worth sparing the same thought for the underwear you wear to a sewing class. If a sewing teacher or fellow student is going to help you with your fitting, they'll likely glimpse your underwear. Now is not the occasion for period pants.

Danger, high risk!

Naked sewing can come with associated risks to sensitive parts of the human body – particularly if you're going bra-less. And bending over the machine. Maybe a comfy T-shirt bra is not such a bad idea, after all... Consider yourself warned!

> 'I was sewing in my underwear to save precious time. All went well until my son walked in with his new girlfriend. Sadly, that relationship didn't last very long – I do hope I wasn't the cause of its early demise.' Blog reader, Tiger Lily

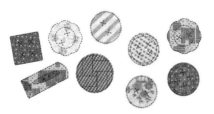

BODY MEASURING TOOLS

Accurate body measurements are key to successful sewing. As well as a clear eye and honest assessment, there are other body measuring tools that will help you create a well-fitting outfit to feel awesome in.

A friend

Some measurements are really difficult to take on your own. Ever tried measuring from the nape of your neck to the base of your spine? Exactly. Get a friend to help and turn it into a fun afternoon with a few nibbles and maybe something bubbly. Sewing can be uber-social!

Close-fitting layers

Wear close-fitting and simple clothes. A gathered skirt and ruffle blouse will only give you inaccurate numbers.

Body measurement table

Once you've taken down your measurements, transfer them to a table that you can refer to whenever you need. You'll find several to download online or in sewing reference books. One option is to draw up your own table in a sewing journal. Lots of sewists use an exercise book to record details of sewing projects, along with fabric swatches, adjustment notes – and body measurements.

Tape measure

Invest in a new one. Vintage tape measures may look pretty, but they were often made from cloth tape that stretches and distorts, giving inaccurate measurements.

When measuring, pull the tape snug but not tight. Make sure the tape doesn't sag around the back of the waist or around your hips. When measuring your chest, the tape should stretch across the apex of your bust. (For apex, read nipples.)

The tip of a standard width tape measure is exactly 15 mm - the same size as a standard seam allowance.

Elastic cord

I love this tip! If you take a length of 1 mm elastic and knot it around your waist, the cord will naturally roll to the slimmest part of your body, helping you identify exactly where your waist is. Some of us have a higher or lower waistline than others and some of us don't have a well-defined waist, so this really helps.

Final note

Your body is constantly changing. This means that you'll need to update your body measurements regularly. Take them for long enough and you'll end up with a surprising journal of your body that beats any online dashboard or training app. For good or bad, I still know what my waist measured ten years ago. It's pencilled in the back of a notebook...

CHOOSING A PATTERN SIZE

You have picked out the sewing pattern of dreams, and now you have your body measurements. How do you know which size to cut out or trace?

These are the four details most important to bear in mind:

- Pattern company size chart

- Finished garment measurements

- Wearing ease

- Personal taste

Pattern company size chart

You'll often find this printed on the envelope flap for the pattern. Typically, it's a chart that shows you columns for bust, waist and hip measurements. Below those there should be a column for your suggested pattern size and below that should be a final column showing you the finished garment measurements.

If you are between sizes, it's recommended that you go up a size rather than down. After all, you can always remove fabric from a make, but you can't add fabric once your pieces have been cut.

Finished measurements

This is the size of the garment, once wearing or design ease has been taken into account. A commercial pattern company typically prints these measurements on the back of the pattern envelope or on the pattern tissue itself. On the pattern tissues, look for a little symbol of a circle with a cross in it – beside it should be the finished garment measurements.

Many experienced sewists swear by checking the finished garment measurements, and fit according to those. They may entirely ignore the sizing suggestions on the pattern envelope as some commercial pattern companies build in a lot of ease – up to 10 centimetres (4 in.).

What is wearing ease?

You know how you like to bend over, eat and sit down without your clothes splitting? Wearing ease allows you to do that. It usually comprises 2.5–5 centimetres (1–2 in.) extra fabric on top of your body measurement to allow your body to squish about inside your outfit as you move. For example, if your waist measurement is 76 centimetres (30 in.), the finished item might have a waist measurement of 81 centimetres (32 in.)

Wearing ease isn't important only for your comfort. It can also make a big difference to design, and how an outfit looks on the body. If something is too tight, it causes wrinkles and bumps. A little extra fabric allows the make to hang smoothly over your body and your hard work won't end up full of creases the first time you bend over.

Trust me, wearing ease is your friend. Use it!

HOW MUCH EASE IS GOOD EASE?

As a general rule, 4-5 centimetres (11/2-2 in.) of ease is great. Anything more than that and your beautiful dress could end up looking like an ill-fitting sack.

Personal taste

Do bear in mind that, with all the above, personal taste enters the mix. You might love a tight-fitting wiggle dress or you may prefer a loose and blousy fit. Know what YOU are comfortable wearing and go with that.

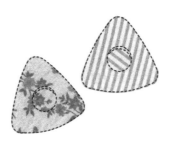

FOOD AND SEWING

Pizza or cheesecake? Prosecco or Aperol Spritz? Ah, food – one of life's great sensual pleasures. But our relationship with food can also be incredibly complex and this has implications for your sewing.

A person can spend weeks slaving over the perfect fit, only to discover six months later that they have gained or lost weight, started an exercise regime or had a health issue – and suddenly that dress doesn't fit any more.

This can be disheartening, but it may also be an opportunity to measure your relationship with food in an objective way, stripping some of the emotion out of what is always a highly emotive topic. When you're forced to disregard outfits you spent weeks sewing, it focuses the mind.

There are some questions you can ask yourself.

- What has changed in the rest of my life between then and now?

- How has this affected my eating habits?

- Can I sew new outfits to suit my new body shape?

- Does it matter if I need to sew new outfits in the future?

- Do I have the skills to address these challenges?

If the answer to the last three questions is a resounding YES, you are on the path to sewing yourself happy. It's really important to employ plenty of self-kindness to yourself at these times. Food is to be enjoyed and so is sewing.

And while we're on the topic of eating, here are some tips for what's going into your gob while your fabric goes under your sewing machine.

Alcohol

One in seven people drink at home. How many of them also sew, that's what I want to know! We all love a tipple, but be careful around alcohol and sewing. Many an outfit has been ruined after one glass too many. Ask me how I know...

Greasy foods

Especially if you're handling delicate fabric, I'd stay away from the kebabs. If you do need to eat greasy foods while sewing, be rigorous about washing your hands after the last morsel has entered your mouth.

Cotton gloves

Depending on how important your make is (wedding dresses, I'm looking at you!) you may even want to wear cotton gloves while sewing your delicate fabrics. Can't say I've ever tried this one myself.

Take a break

When you're sewing to a deadline (it happens, sometimes) it's easy to enter a seven-hour sewing marathon and forget to do the essential things in life, like eat. It's really important to step away from the machine and refuel. If nothing else, this allows you to rest your brain. With your mind and body back to operating at their best, you're less likely to make mistakes.

FITTING TECHNIQUES

Once you've chosen your pattern size, it's time to start fitting. You might be impatient to launch straight into your make, cutting out expensive fashion fabric. The danger is that you'll come up against a fitting challenge and your lovely fabric that you've spent many an evening stroking (don't worry, we all do it) ends up in the bin.

There are ways to avoid disappointment.

Tissue fitting

This is a technique where you pin your paper patter pieces together and 'try on' your 3-D outfit in tissue paper. I was the world's worst cynic about this technique but it works.

How do you tissue fit?

- Trace your pattern pieces or work with the original tissue pieces.

- Apply masking tape around curves such as armholes to protect them from splitting.

- Pencil in seam allowances.

- Fold darts and pleats into place and pin through the paper.

- Pin seams together, so that the seam allowance sits on the outside.

- Don't try to pin together the whole make – test a bodice or skirt piece separately.

- Carefully 'try on' your pinned piece and assess for adjustment.

- Pinch out any baggy sections or mark up places where the pattern may need to be cut and spread.

A toile

A toile (or muslin) is a practice make using either calico or a cheap fabric of a similar weight and drape to your chosen fashion fabric. This allows you to test the fit of an outfit and make any final adjustments before launching into the final make. It also allows you to:

- Assess how the outfit looks on you

- Adjust any design elements such as collar width or hem length

- Practice tricky techniques

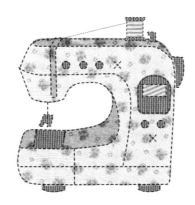

HOW DO YOU SEW A TOILE?

- Choose a suitable and inexpensive fabric.
- Cut out your pattern pieces, taking on board any adjustments you've made at the tissue fitting stage.
- Sew up the toile pieces using a long tacking stitch for speed and quick ripping out if needed.
- Use a contrasting thread for ease of spotting fit adjustments.
- Mark up any changes on your fabric.
- Don't worry about making a mess – toiles are messy.
- Don't blanche at how unflattering the toile looks – the whole point of a toile is that there's nowhere to hide fit issues.
- Transfer any adjustments to your paper pattern pieces.
- You're done!

Struggling with fit?

Recruit Online Friends: The great thing about an online sewing community is that you have free access to a wealth of expertise. If you have the humility to post photos of a badly fitting item, you're guaranteed to receive tips and wisdom from people with a lifetime's experience and expertise. Reach out!

Attend A Sewing Class: Sewing classes don't only encourage you to improve your skills: they often afford you access to teachers with decades of sewing experience and an extra pair of hands to help you fit an item. The number one reason people attend sewing classes is to help them fit.

Study Online: There is a raft of learning-from-home e-courses that can help you with fit. Craftsy is the number one platform, but you can also enjoy video tutorials from Threads online and YouTube.

Book Resources: Here are some well-loved books on fitting:

- *Pattern Fitting with Confidence*, Nancy Zieman

- *Fit for Real People*, Pati Palmer and Marta Alto

- *Fitting and Pattern Alteration*, Elizabeth L Liechty, Della N Pottberg-Steineckert and Judith A Rasband

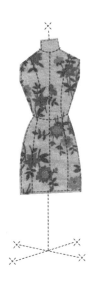

EVERY BODY'S WONKY

'A university professor set my theatrical costuming class this conundrum: "How many darts does it take to cover a hump?" We were costuming Richard III.'
Blog reader, Lin

The point is, every body is different. Very different. I'm setting you a challenge:

- Go and get naked. (I know, again!)

- Now, stand in front of a full-length mirror.

- Once you've stopped laughing, turn around on the spot and look at yourself from different angles.

What do you see? I see...

- A left shoulder that's lower than the right shoulder. That's why I always have a bra strap slipping off one shoulder.

- A huge scar running up my tummy from a myomectomy.

- That my face isn't symmetrical. (Whose is?) That's why sunglasses always sit at an angle.

- The start of a dowager's hump. Dowager's hump. Two of the ugliest words in the world.

There are over 7 billion people in the world. That's 7 billion different bodies - every one unique. And if all those people sewed, that would be 7 billion different fitting challenges.

Once you put it like that, it's hard to beat yourself up.

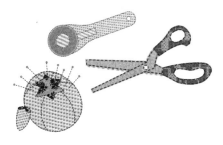

SEXUALITY AND SEWING

'Hey girl, can I just say that you quilting all day long in your pyjamas is... so SEXY.'

Internet meme

During my time sewing, I have seen women dare to be sexy again, transgender people experiment with fashion choices, drag queens set up with outrageous costumes and teenagers sew their first romantic prom dresses.

Sex and sewing – it's a journey!

Sewing is full of secrets; that's why it's so gorgeous. Satin, silk, chiffon, lace... We've got it all going on. From secretly lining a dress with silk to sewing your own decadent kimono, running up a bombshell swimsuit, picking out vintage lace to decorate your décolletage or sewing a perfectly tailored men's shirt... sewing and sex is a win-win.

I've lost count of the number of sewing blogs where a sewist coyly states, 'My partner really liked this make...' There's a lot of fun to be had, but my guess is that most people sew for themselves first.

They're happy, and that makes other people happy. They're confident, and confidence is sexy. Before you know it, you're knocking people dead in the street when you popped out for a bottle of milk!

Being sexy isn't just about what you wear, it's about how you feel. And sewing makes you feel good!

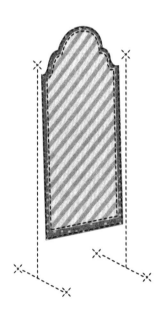

COMMON FITTING
ADJUSTMENTS

There are a few fitting adjustments that people come across time and again. Once you have become familiar with the demands of your own body shape, there are certain techniques that you will confidently be able to get under your belt and whip out whenever they're needed.

Lengthening or shortening

One of the first dresses I made didn't fit. Fabric pooled around the waist and I couldn't work out what was happening. I took photos and sent out a request to my online friends. What was wrong? It turned out the adjustment was really simple: my bodice pieces were too long.

Most often, people need to shorten or lengthen either a bodice, a skirt or arm pieces – sometimes all three.

Most commercial patterns have adjustment lines marked for lengthening or shortening. It's advisable to make your adjustments where marked, as these shall allow you to keep intact the shape of the finished garment. For example, if you're making a tulip skirt you don't want to lop 5 centimetres (2 in.) off the hem – not without distorting that pretty tulip shape.

Look for those adjustment lines!

Bust adjustment

Ever pulled on a dress that fits across the chest but is voluminous around the arms and shoulders? Or do you have a small bust for your size and find this part of your outfit bagging?

Most high-street clothes use standard measurements that don't allow for the fact that a woman can be large of chest and narrow of shoulders, or have wide shoulders and a small bust or… well, any variation from an out-of-date set of mean statistics. By mean, I mean average but I could mean… oh, you know what I mean!

Moving on.

Fortunately, sewing allows you to tweak for a perfect chest fit. The Full or Small Bust Adjustment involves cutting out a pattern to the sizing on your upper chest. You then trace and cut lines leading to the bust point and either spread or overlap the pattern piece.

For detailed instructions on either a Full or Small Bust Adjustment, you'll find lots of tutorials online and in sewing books. These techniques look scary, but I promise you they're not once you've familiarized yourself – and then your fitting life will be changed forever.

Moving dart tips

Oh yes, those curves are coming in to play again. Guess what? Women's boobs aren't all the same size and shape. No kidding, right?

This means that dart placements in a bodice often need to be adjusted according to the demands of your body. Your body changes over time, so this is a fitting detail that you should regularly check.

The type of bra you wear can also make a significant difference, so be sure to wear the same bra during fitting as you'll wear with the finished make.

To raise or lower a bust dart – the most common dart that needs adjusting – simply hold the front bodice pattern piece against your chest and mark where your apex (nipple) sits against the pattern piece. If this is significantly higher or lower than the point of the dart, you'll need to move the dart placement on your pattern piece accordingly.

I've found lots of pretty complex-looking online tutorials for moving a bust dart. Honestly, I usually just slide the original paper pattern piece down or up to where I need the new dart positioning and trace the dart there, being sure to retain the original length of the bodice. Shoot me down in flames if you like! It works for me.

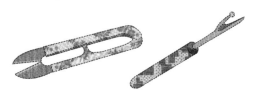

YOUR CHANGING BODY

As you move through life, your body changes. Sometimes we choose these changes. These can be times of happiness, but they can also be times of anxiety. Sewing allows us to accommodate these changes - we find our new selves at the end of a tape measure.

Adolescence

We don't all grow at the same rate. Some of us shoot up and out, others take longer. Stretch marks, acne, trainer bras, changing voice - it's a joy and a minefield. But it only happens once.

Pregnancy

Wow, so this is a change, huh? Difficult to predict how it will affect you - high bump, low bump, swelling breasts, raging hormones, shortness of breath. Will you even be able to sew in the final trimester? On the plus side, cute baby clothes to make!

Menopause

For women entering the menopause, this can be a testing time. Everything you've taken to be true about your body starts to change. Some of the signs that affect our sewing include a thickening torso, flatter derrière and lower bust.

Gender reassignment

If this is you, you're learning about your body all over again, with a whole raft of details that you never even knew about. New underwear, new body shape – do you even know what style you like to wear? How do you find clothes to fit? Do they make you feel masculine or feminine and how does that matter to you? This is where sewing really comes into its own! If you aren't confident to sew your own new wardrobe, or need help fitting, you can find a tailor or seamstress who specializes in working with the transgender community. Or find a friend who sews!

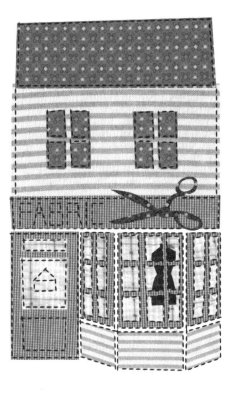

CHAPTER 4

MENTAL HEALTH

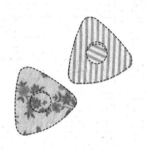

Mindfulness, being in the moment, zen meditation – sewing is all of these and so much more. If you've ever dealt with anxiety or stress, suffered panic attacks or found yourself unable to sleep, you're probably already aware of the benefits of a repetitive, meditative activity... an activity like sewing. I'm not suggesting you get up in the night to sew (though who am I to judge), but if you factor meditative sewing into your day, you may reduce anxiety.

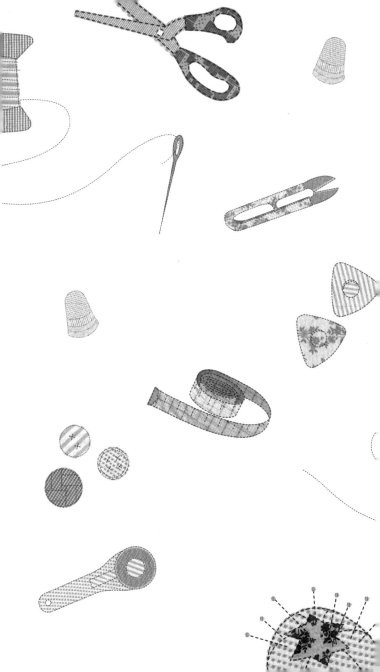

Sew yourself calm

Mindful sewing

Conquer your biggest sewing fears

How to read a sewing pattern

Tidy sewing, tidy mind

Wrestling the worm of sewing doubt

Ten reasons why sewing is good for your
mental health

You will learn:
To conquer the machine buttonhole
First tailoring tips
How to read a sewing pattern
How to use fusible interfacing

SEW YOURSELF CALM

The world can feel like a crazy place sometimes. Who am I kidding? The world can feel like a crazy place a lot of the time. Rolling news, social media, multi-tasking, deskbound day jobs, open-plan offices, four-hour commutes, babies, careers, having it all, not having it all... Phewee.

Whenever I've found myself feeling hopeless and helpless in the face of world events or situations out of my control, I turn to sewing. Typically, I turn to a small, specific sewing task that demands my full concentration for a limited amount of time. It's my sewing equivalent of a 20-minute session with a meditation app.

Typical acts of sewing meditation could be:

- Tracing a pattern
- Hand stitching a hem
- Pinning a sleeve insertion
- Cutting out fabric

Other helpful tips for sewing meditation:

- A familiar-to-you technique
- A fresh brain
- A quiet room
- Switching off the phone and laptop

Twenty minutes later, anger is forgotten and stress has dissolved away. It works every time. And you're closer to another finished sewing project. What's not to love?

MINDFUL SEWING

'An important part of mindfulness is reconnecting with our bodies and the sensations they experience. This means waking up to the sights, sounds, smells and tastes of the present moment.'
Professor Mark Williams, Oxford Medical Centre

What is mindfulness? It's a peaceful mental state achieved by being in the moment. When this comes to sewing it might involve:

- Guiding a thread through a needle

- Listening to the snip of scissors through fabric

- Judging the right colour of thread for your project

- Sewing on an appliqué patch

- Machine darning a hole in your jeans

If you want this mindfulness to carry on through the make you might consider:

- Sewing a secret message in a collar or yoke

- Repeating a positive mantra as you sew

- Choosing a fabric print for its symbolism or colours that comfort you

- Moving your sewing outside for a full sensory overload (if it's sunny!)

- Working in silence

SEWING FEARS

'I'm terrified of sewing collars! When I was 13 years old, I took a sewing course and the only thing I didn't learn was to insert collars! I'm 29 years old now, and I've never made a top with a collar.'

Blog reader, Mia

It's true. There's a lot about sewing that can seem scary. Believe me, there are techniques I still avoid. But you're not alone and if we're going to tackle those fears, we need to name them. Over the page are some of the most common fears that sewists face. Do you recognize any?

Fitting

Fear: I hate it when things don't fit when I've spent ages making it or spent loads of money on the fabric and notions! In fact, this exact fear is what makes me seriously lose my sewing mojo!

Answer: Online message boards, reference books and blogs can help, but teaching yourself at home can only take you so far. My advice is to go to a sewing class and access an experienced tutor. They'll be able to help you understand why something doesn't fit and help you fix that.

Wasting time

Fear: Wasting time on something that ends up being a wadder. I have very little free time, so I absolutely hate wasting my sewing time on something I can't wear.

Answer: There is no such thing as wasted sewing time. Easy for me to say, I know! But sewing is like running, writing or giving birth (okay, maybe not like giving birth) – it's a muscle that needs exercising. When someone is writing a novel, deleting thousands of words along the way, they're not wasting time. They're learning. So are you.

Buttonholes

Fear: Buttonholes are my nemesis.

Answer: Buttonholes are scary. They are often one of the last steps in a make and they involve slicing open fabric. It can also be easy to get buttonholes wrong and then they're tricky to unpick. Here's how to avoid that:

- Add a patch of fusible interfacing to the wrong side of your fabric.

- Does your bobbin case have a hole in the arm? Thread your bobbin thread through this to improve the stitch tension of a buttonhole.

- Test your buttonhole stitching on a swatch first.

- Make sure there is enough fabric under your sewing machine foot so that the teeth can grip and move your make. There's nothing worse than a buttonhole that gets stuck.

- Use a chisel rather than a seam ripper to open up your buttonhole.

- A few drops of Fray Check shall stop your buttonholes unravelling.

- An expanding buttonhole gauge is lots of fun and allows for accurate spacing of buttonholes.

- Relax and have fun!

Wasting fabric

Fear: Cutting into a treasured piece of fabric. What if it doesn't fit and the fabric is wasted?

Answer: Ask yourself this: did you buy that fabric for it to sit in a drawer for the next ten years? Of course not. Repeat after me. It's only fabric, it's only fabric… What's the worst that can happen? If you do find that you've wasted fabric on a make that doesn't work, see my suggestions for recycling a make on page 216.

The seam ripper

Fear: Slipping with the seam ripper. That blade is sharp!

Answer: A seam ripper is a small tool with a curved blade for ripping out stitches, but go too far and you could tear the fabric on your make. To avoid this, place a pin in your fabric at the place you want to stop ripping. You'll never rip an ugly hole again.

Tailoring

Fear: I'm afraid of making jackets. Don't ask me why, but I have countless patterns, fabric and lining ready to go – but for some reason I will not start the project.

Answer: Entering the world of tailoring usually

heralds a step up in your sewing. It's not surprising that fear of failure makes some people freeze in the headlights. But if you take things one step at a time and gather your arsenal – equipment, supplies and learning tools – you'll find you can achieve more than you ever dreamt of and tailor a jacket or coat from scratch. Yes, you! One of my first projects was a coat sewn from cashmere wool and I've never looked back.

- ◉ Source decent tailoring supplies – see the Resources section on page 220.

- ◉ Buy, steal or borrow a copy of *The Reader's Digest Guide To Sewing*.

- ◉ Choose a simple pattern for your first make. Kimono jackets and cocoon coats are relatively easy.

- ◉ Pick out a colour to make your heart sing – you won't be able to resist sewing.

- Have fun with lining fabric. You can play with a bold print or bright colour.

- Break the process down into small, digestible steps.

- Plan the timing. If you want a winter coat, start in the autumn. It sounds obvious, but you'd be amazed how many summers I've spent sewing with hot wool.

- Lap up the compliments when you have finished. Yes, I made this!

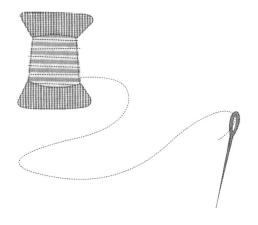

HOW TO READ A
SEWING PATTERN

Research shows that learning through life improves a person's happiness, optimism and mental health. So, are you ready to learn how a set of sewing pattern instructions works?

Typically, these come in two or even three sheets, printed in black and white and folded inside the pattern envelope. Some indie pattern companies might supply a full-colour booklet but by and large, instructions follow the same format.

Pattern envelope

- Sizing table – to judge fabric requirements

- Technical illustration

- Suggested fabrics

- Notions – what extra resources you'll need to buy, such as elastic or zips

🔘 Body measurements and finished
measurement table (see page 70)

Instruction sheets

Technical Illustrations: These show you the design lines of the finished garment. Take a moment to look at them, as they will help you understand the construction.

Pattern Symbols Key: They may look like hieroglyphics, but they're there to help you put the pattern together properly. Some of the most common are:

Pattern Pieces: A line drawing of each pattern piece, each of them cross-referenced to a label, to help you identify all the pieces printed on your tissue or paper.

Fabric and Cutting Layouts: This bird's-eye diagram shows you how to arrange the pattern pieces on your fabric for cutting out. I don't always follow these suggestions, but they are a decent guide, especially if you're using a directional print.

WHAT IS A DIRECTIONAL PRINT?

This is where the print on a fabric all faces the same way - for example, Christmas trees all in a row. You'll need to take note of a directional print when cutting out fabric to ensure that you don't end up with upside-down Christmas trees on your dress, or certain pieces where the design has flipped.

General Instructions: These will give you guidelines, such as letting you know if fabric needs prewashing (yes, always!) and a few other basic rules of sewing.

Glossary of Terminology: This allows you to understand any unfamiliar language in the instructions.

Sewing Instructions: Along with illustrations, ideally these instructions should be easy to follow. I say, ideally. Some can be pretty dense and take user knowledge for granted. In reaction to this, there has been a recent surge in independent pattern companies looking to provide easy-to-use and clear pattern instructions. If you get stuck at any point, I recommend going to blogs or websites such as The Foldline or Sewing Pattern Review for hints and tips from other sewists who often flag tricky stages and how to negotiate them.

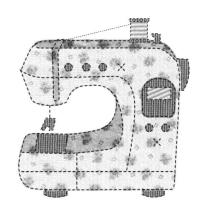

TIDY SEWING, TIDY MIND

There are no rules to creativity. Some people love working in chaos; others need a clean and minimalist space. Even if your sewing room looks as though a bomb's gone off by the end of a project, I recommend making your process tidy. It will really help you keep your sewing on course.

Cutting out

Do all your cutting out – fashion fabric, lining and interfacing – at the same time. There is nothing worse than having to drag the cutting mat back out because you forgot to cut out those two pocket pieces. It's a bore and a chore and the sooner you get all the cutting out of the way, the sooner you can start sewing.

Notching and tacks

When you cut out your pieces, you'll see little triangles on the cutting-out line. This is where you should snip notches into your seam allowance, to help you line up pattern pieces. You might also see places marked with a small solid dot on the pattern pieces for the placement of tailor's tacks. Do all your notching and tailor's tacks before sewing commences. I promise, it's a timesaver.

WHAT IS A TAILOR'S TACK?

This is a tacking stitch that uses a double length of thread to mark positions on a pattern piece. They're often used to help you transfer markings from paper pattern pieces onto your fashion fabric. They help with the placement of darts, pleats, pockets and other construction details. They don't leave marks on the fabric and are easily removed.

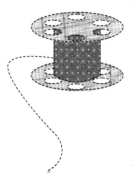

FUSIBLE INTERFACING TIPS

- Buy good quality interfacing - see Resources section on page 220.
- Keep your iron on a moderate heat and use a press cloth to avoid melting your interfacing.
- When moving the iron, pick it up and press it back down on a new section of interfacing. Don't glide your iron across, as this shall cause ripples in the interfacing.
- Match the colour of your interfacing to your fashion fabric - white or neutral interfacing for light colours, black interfacing for darker colours.
- If you are interfacing sections that will be sliced open, such as buttonholes, be aware that the interfacing may peek through.

Fuse your fabric

Immediately after cutting out, add any fusible interfacing to the relevant pattern pieces. Again, if you do this at the start of the process it will save you unnecessary headaches once you're deep in the sewing.

Gather your pattern pieces

Remove all pins from your cut-out pattern pieces. If you leave pins in your fabric, you run the danger of permanent puncture marks. You can leave one pin to keep pattern piece and tissue paper together (this helps identify pattern pieces as you turn to them), but make sure the pin sits inside a seam allowance.

Then gather your cut out pieces in one place so that they are easy to find as you work through your project.

Prepare your machine

How often do you clean your sewing machine? It's worth doing this before each new project – dusting off the moving parts, cleaning out the throat plate and feed dog, changing the needle and oiling the hook race. Your machine should come with a manual to help you do this.

Find a natural pause

When you step away from the sewing – hey, we've all got to sleep! – try to leave the work as you finish a technique step. It can be a real head scratcher to pick something up after a few days and try to remember what you were doing.

Put equipment away

I try to put equipment away once I've finished using it. The cutting mat goes back behind the sideboard, scissors are returned to the sewing basket after use, the ironing board is folded up at the end of a session. Yes, you may end up pulling those scissors back out, but this helps you feel in control of your sewing.

Who says sewing can't be zen!

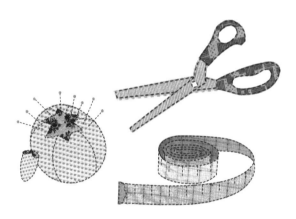

WRESTLING THE WORM OF SEWING DOUBT

I cannot tell a lie. There are moments during a sewing project when the worm of self-doubt wriggles to the surface. As with all creative pursuits, this is inevitable at some stage. The good news is that there are concrete ways to bash that worm into submission.

Step away

If doubt starts to cloud your judgement, it's a good idea to step away from the work. Ten times out of ten, a good night's sleep helps you come back to a project with clarity and perspective. Maybe you're just too tired to sew.

Reach out

I've said it before and I'll say it again – there's no community like the sewing community. Put a call out on social media and there will be people all around the world willing to help put your mind at rest or confirm your worst fears. Either way, they'll help you come up with a solution.

Re-read the instructions

Skipping instructions is easy to do. It can also mean you miss crucial details. If a step just doesn't make sense, make yourself a drink and sit down with the instructions. You may discover that you've missed a key detail.

Choose a manageable task

You don't always have to follow the sequence of sewing instructions for a project. If you're feeling overwhelmed by a key stage, why not skip forwards to a more manageable task such as making pockets, finishing seams or staystitching a neckline? You'll have an activity that makes you feel productive and in control, allowing you to return to the bigger tasks with a fresh and more confident mind.

Stop sewing

Sewing should be a pleasure, not a chore. If you're not enjoying it, stop. Take a few days off. When you're ready, you'll come back to it. Some of the best thinking time takes place when you're doing something totally mindless - walking the dog, cleaning your teeth, mowing the lawn. Even in your dreams, your sewing eureka moment may strike.

TEN REASONS WHY SEWING IS GOOD FOR YOUR MENTAL HEALTH

- It gives you dedicated time for yourself.

- Sewing releases dopamine in the brain. The dopamine hormone is linked to pleasure.

- Time at the sewing machine gives you a digital detox, taking you away from electronic devices.

- You learn new skills – and learning new skills is one way of lessening the threat of dementia.

- It's a new source of self-esteem – it's important not to ground all your sense of self in one channel.

- Mindful sewing allows you to live in the moment.

- Sewing gives you a sense of achievement.

- It also gives you cool new clothes!

- You prove your unique place in the world. No one else made what you just made.

- It can be your go-to coping strategy for stress.

Still not convinced? Then turn to our next chapter and find out how sewing can make you a kinder person...

CHAPTER 5

KINDNESS

'One of the best gifts is my mom's help. We muslined jeans for me and now I make jeans that fit me. We went shopping many years ago and I tried on over 50 pairs of trousers to find a single pair that fit. Now I can cut and sew a pair in two days.'

Blog reader, Chris

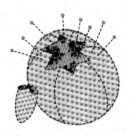

Kindness matters more than ever.
The modern world connects us through
social media, rolling news, blogs and vlogs.
We see lives other than our own, which is
great for building our empathy skills.
But if those lives take place on the other side
of a screen, it can be easy to disassociate or
idealise. That person with the perfect life
surely doesn't need me,
or my approval.

But we do. We need each other. The world
can be a scary place and it's up to us to
show empathy and, yes, kindness. And
not just to help others – science proves
that a single kind act releases serotonin,
endorphins and oxytocin.

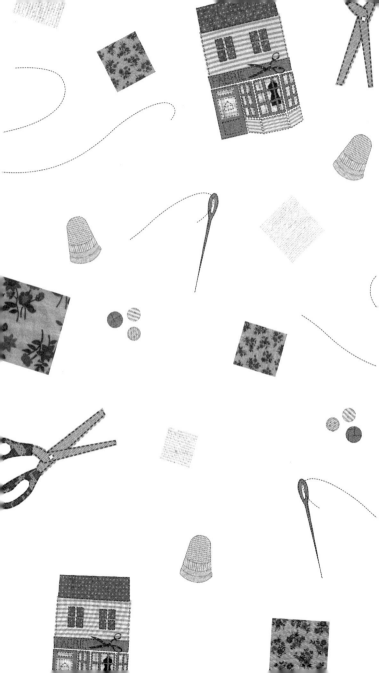

Communication

How to choose fabrics

A silver thimble

Q&A with sewing friends

Sewing when it counts

Sewing scissors

Cutting out fabric

Be kind to your fabric

You will learn:

How to choose fabric

The best sewing scissors

How to cut out pattern pieces

Fabric care

COMMUNICATION

Do you consider yourself to be a dressmaker or a seamstress? A sewist or a maker? There are lots of different words for our hobby. Words matter.

They matter especially when we are feeding back on each other's makes. Sometimes we're feeding back in real life; often this engagement takes place online. It's important to be kind, inclusive and considerate in our choice of words.

Emojis are your friend

No, they're not silly. Emojis help us communicate with each other. They've even made it into the *Oxford English Dictionary*. Cracking a joke? Add a 'laughing' emoji. Want to defuse an argument? Add a 'laughing so hard I'm crying' emoji. Emojis give us emotional framing for online conversations. They do all the work of tone of voice, facial expressions and gestures. So be kind to yourself and others, and litter your comments with emojis! Seriously.

Body shape

If we're commenting on another person's sewing, we're not commenting on their body shape or even what we perceive to be flattering. Remember, aesthetics are personal. Keep body language out of it and focus on the awesome achievement.

The nuance of language

There are some words and phrases that I try to avoid around sewing discussions online:

- Lovely – an author friend flagged the danger of telling female professionals they're lovely. It lacks content. Now I try to avoid the word in all my feedback to, well, anyone.

- Pretty – a longstanding rule of mine to avoid praising children only by their looks. Should we apply the same rule to our adult friends?

- Girlpower – I'm not a girl, but I am powerful.

- Selfish sewing – it doesn't make you selfish to sew for yourself.

- Gender specific – I try to ensure that any blog post I write could be read by either men, women or transgender people. Sewing is not a female-only pursuit.

I'm sure you'll have your own words you try to avoid.

Follow hashtags

If you want to make it clear what your photo represents, what you stand for and what language you will tolerate from others, a hashtag can go a long way:

- #bodyconfidence

- #plussizesewing

- #lovetheskinyouarein

- #kindnessmatters

Finally.

If you don't have anything good to say... don't say it. It's a simple rule, but it works.

HOW TO CHOOSE FABRICS

'With these dainty, colourful and durable fabrics, you can make the most lovely frocks, dresses and undies for your Spring and Summer wear!'
Woman's Magazine, April 1939

Learning how to choose the right fabric for your make is one of the never-ending lessons of sewing. Sewists only learn by experience and early mistakes are inevitable. You can still make unfortunate choices after decades of sewing, but here are my tips to help you choose the perfect fabric to work with your pattern.

When you're about to indulge that impulse purchase, here is a handy checklist for making sure you're splurging on perfection!

Machine washable

Can you toss your fabric into the washing machine on a 40-degree wash? Yes, if we're caring for the environment we wash at 30 degrees – but sometimes we crank it up, and sometimes we forget that our precious handmade dress might not survive a hotter cycle. Oops!

If you know that you hate going to the dry cleaners or always forget to use the Delicate Wash cycle, it might be worth pausing to consider if your new fabric will survive the washing machine.

Wool needs dry cleaning, viscose can shrink, linen fades and silk may need a hand wash.

Think realistically about how you launder your makes.

A cohesive wardrobe

Before buying three metres of a rather special print, try to imagine it with other items that already exist in your wardrobe. If you can't, does this mean you'll need to make or buy other items to create a cohesive wardrobe? Do you want to? Great, if you do. If you're less sure, you might want to put that bolt of fabric back on the shelf.

What do you already wear?

When you're shopping for clothes, do you tend to buy jersey or cotton, silk or cupro? What you buy in your ready-made wardrobe may help you decide what fabrics to choose. Do you wear solids or colours? Structural dresses or floaty blouses? If you never wear jeans, is it worth buying denim? When 90 per cent of your shop-bought clothes are jersey, should you really buy that cotton?

Hate ironing?

Hey, I feel ya! It's a big consideration, especially when choosing fabrics. I often take a corner of the bolt and crunch it up in my hand to watch how the fabric then releases. If it creases easily, I might put it back. Great fabrics for avoiding creases are polyester, crepe, wool, poplin cotton and high-quality cotton lawn. Great fabric for embracing creases is linen!

Check the pattern envelope

Each sewing pattern should come with fabric suggestions on the pattern envelope. Not only will these guide you as to the weight and drape of fabric, they can also steer you away from directional prints or stripes that might be difficult to accommodate in the pattern design. The pattern envelope will also tell you how much fabric to buy, but as a general rule:

- 1.5 metres (1⅝ yd) = a top or blouse

- 2 metres (2¼ yd) = a slim-fitting dress

- 3 metres (3¼ yd) = trousers or a dress with lots of gathers or detail

- 4 metres (4⅜ yd) = a coat or other large project

Don't forget that fabric width also impacts on how much fabric to buy. Fabric comes in a variety of widths, but the most common are 90 centimetres, 119 centimetres and 150 centimetres (36, 46 and 60 in.). If in doubt, I usually buy 2 metres (2¼ yd) of fabric. If I want to be on the safe side, I buy 3 metres (3¼ yd).

Solid or print?

Ah, the great debate. Do you love a colourful print or might you prefer the pared-down palette of a capsule wardrobe? Both have their place. It's worth sparing time to work with solid colours, because these can be striking, adaptable go-to items in your wardrobe that will be worn again and again. And if you really want to see the design lines of a sewing project, then solid colours will create the best platform. On the other hand, busy prints are magnificent at hiding mistakes! Your call.

Natural or synthetic?

- If you're shopping online, read the fabric description.

- If you're buying in a fabric shop, look at the label on the end of the bolt.

- If you're buying on a market, cross your fingers!

Once you start sewing, you realize how important the composition of a fabric is. You may prefer breathable fabrics in order to accommodate your body temperature – though do remember that natural fabrics require the press of an iron. Alternatively, you may choose something you can toss in a suitcase, in which case seek out polyesters. Each fabric comes with its pros and cons, so decide what's important to you.

A SILVER THIMBLE

*'My luxury would be a thimble. I use a
tailor's thimble... it's one of those things I
work with every day, I need it. When I get
up in the morning I put my thimble on
like I put my clothes on, it's part of me...
I'm going to give it to you, though.'*

Milliner Philip Treacy to presenter
Kirsty Young, Desert Island Discs

The sewing accoutrements we gather around us
come to represent so much more than sewing...

Theo and I met at a time in my life when I was
stressed and overwhelmed. But we shared a love of
dogs and walking, and he was my release. For our
first Christmas, he presented me with a little gold
box that contained a vintage silver thimble. I was
incredibly touched by how thoughtful the gift was.
Two months later, we split up.

I still have that little gold box and I still use the
thimble, the silver etched with daisies. Every time
I settle down to an extended period of hand stitching, I gather my arsenal. Thread, beeswax, my

little felt needle book, pincushion… thimble. Hand sewing is an intensely meditative act. It requires a lamp, something to binge watch or listen to, a glass of something cold and dry. It also requires you to empty your brain and concentrate on the act in hand. The hiss of thread passing through fabric, the glint of a needle as it punctures the warp or weft, the see-sawing motion of your hand, the silence, the patience, the halo of light. A little dog's warm flank pressed against your thigh.

I still think about Theo every time I bring out that thimble. I'm sure he's long forgotten me, or the fact that he ever bought a silver thimble. But I still have it and whenever that silver thimble glows in the lamplight, it reminds me to be kind to myself.

The longer you sew, the more memories you gather. Some life lessons, too.

Q&A WITH SEWING FRIENDS

There's no friend like a sewing friend – it's true! Friendship has always been incredibly important in my life and I think this is part of the reason I'm so drawn to sewing – I just love the people. I always say I've never met a sewist I didn't like. Here's a rundown of the best questions to ask a sewing friend...

Does my bum look big?

Sewing friends never pass comment on bodies. And if your bum is straining your dress, they'll help you work out how to accommodate your toosh. Bodies aren't problems when you're with a sewing pal; they're a technical challenge to be conquered.

Do I need this?

Are you kidding? You always need more fabric. We are here to enable each other and we never pass judgement. Go on - buy another metre to be on the safe side!

Shopping splurge?

You'll never find a sewist in the world who isn't ready, willing and able to join you on a shopping trip. I've even travelled halfway across the world on holiday and still found people to go fabric shopping with me - pals I've never met before. If you can't drag someone along in person, just share the trip in your Instagram stories. They'll help you choose your fabrics if you poll!

Last minute sewing?

Of course you can! Sewists never say 'no', they always say 'Go for it!'.

HOW TO FIND YOUR SEWING TRIBE

If you don't have a sewing friend who lives nearby,
I recommend the following:

- Join an online forum such as The Foldline.
- Take part in an online sewalong like #memademay.
- Tag along on a sewing meet-up – always so much fun!
- Follow hashtags on social media and join in the conversation.
- Ask around in the workplace – I promise you, there'll be someone who sews. .
- Hang out and chat in sewing shops.
- Check out your local noticeboard.
- Do what I did and set up a sewing blog! Or set up a blog, vlog or podcast with a pal.

SEWING WHEN IT COUNTS

There are times in life when others need our kindness or we need to be kind to ourselves. Here are some ideas for spreading the love and kindness of sewing through every stage in life.

House warming

My mum sewed place mats for my sister when she moved to Singapore twenty years ago. My sister has been back in the UK for a long time now, but she still uses those place mats and I still love seeing them every time I visit my her house.

Baby blankets

Those pieces I've made for babies have remained my most often cherished makes. I thought I was making something for a baby, but in a new parent's tired eye these become lifelong keepsakes of a time they'll want to remember – one day! A baby blanket can be a really quick and easy piece of sewing and there are a gazillion tutorials on the Internet. Just try to make your blanket in time for the baby's arrival! I still have quilting squares sat in my sewing box for a baby who's now a toddler.

Grief quilts

I have heard some unbelievably touching stories of quilts that are made using fabric from a loved one's clothes. Obviously, this is an act of kindness and creativity that requires enormous tact, but it can also be incredibly healing for the family who receives it.

Wedding dress

I'm kidding! No, I'm not. I know some people who taught themselves to sew in order to make a wedding dress for their best friend. It happens, people. You can take on this challenge – if you're a braver person than me.

Sewing toys

My grandma made toys for all of her grandchildren and I love seeing home-sewn dolls at craft fairs. There are some wonderful kits and tutorials on the market (I recommend While She Naps as a resource) and this is the ultimate in personalized gifting for the child - or adult! - in your life.

Cancer

There are some fantastic sewing initiatives aimed at helping people when cancer becomes part of their lives. If a friend is ill, it's worth asking if there's anything you can do to help with your sewing. Someone I know lost her hair to treatment and her scalp became very sensitive. I sewed her a hat using the softest cashmere wool I could find. And the kindness passed down the chain - the shop owner helped me choose the best fabric, once she knew what it was for. Kindness can be quiet, but it can also be essential at times like these.

Showing love

Some of us struggle with putting our love into words; others find it difficult to accept large shows of emotion. But if you sew a gift for someone, so much can be said in a small way. You don't even have to make a big show of handing your gift over – just leave it somewhere it can be found.

Sewing self-esteem

Whenever I have found myself feeling low or discouraged, I've turned to sewing. Remember to be kind to yourself, as well as to others.

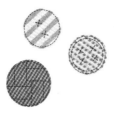

SEWING SCISSORS

*'Pinking Shears Cut Like This /\/\/\/\/\
Save Time And Money With
Pinkrite Pinking Shears!'*
Woman's Magazine, April 1939

Investing in a decent pair of scissors is one of the best acts of kindness you can show yourself if you're taking your sewing career seriously. They will make your life so much easier and happier! If you can't cut out fabric or thread with one efficient – snip! – of blades slicing across each other, you are going to get frustrated quickly.

It goes without saying that you should never use your sewing scissors on anything other than fabric. Hide them from family and friends and give your tersest orders – Not To Be Borrowed. These are mine. Oh, the delicious pleasure of having one item in the house that no one is allowed to use other than their owner. Talk about marking your territory.

Since my early days sewing, I have gathered

quite an arsenal of sewing scissors (fifteen at the last count) and these are what I recommend.

Dressmaking shears

Everyone needs a big, hefty pair of dressmaker's scissors with a nice, long blade. These are sharp enough and long enough to make cutting through fabric like slicing through butter. Remember to open your scissors as wide as they can go to take one long snip. No point pecking away like a baby bird with only the tips of these beautiful scissors.

Pinking shears

The little zig-zag edge of these scissors can be used to finish raw seams – you'll often spot this finishing technique in vintage clothes. Overlockers (sergers) have overtaken pinking scissors as the domestic seam finish of choice, but a pair of pinking shears still comes in useful for finishing the edge of fusible interfacings and hard edges of facings that you don't want to show on the right side of a make.

Rotary cutter

Not a pair of scissors, but a circular blade on a handle. If you use this, combined with a cutting mat, you'll be able to cut out fabric in one long and accurate motion. This is particularly useful for stretch fabrics, floaty fabrics or cutting out accurate quilting squares – anything that won't benefit from the snip, snip, snip of scissors. Be sure to change your blade regularly.

Embroidery scissors

Perfect for snipping the ends of thread. Consider hanging a pair on a length of velvet rope and drape around your neck for the full-on Phantom Thread effect.

Serrated scissors

Ooh, these are a game changer when it comes to cutting out silk or other drapey fabrics. The tiny serrated teeth grip the fabric, which prevents it from billowing away as you cut. This is important for accuracy and sanity.

Left-handed scissors

If you're left handed, like me, you might consider investing in a pair of left-handed scissors. I promise, you don't know what you're missing out on. For the first time in your life, you'll be cutting with the sharp blade!

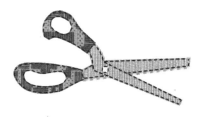

WEIGHING IT UP

If you have weak wrists or other issues with your hands, you might want to avoid the heavier scissors. Choose a lightweight, ergonomic option instead, such as the Singer Professional Series or the Fiskars Easy Action Razor Edge Scissors. Online retailers should provide the weight of scissors in their item descriptions.

CUTTING OUT FABRIC

One of our biggest pleasures is choosing and buying fabric, so it only makes sense to treat it well once it's in our sewing room. If you want to be kind to your fabric, it all starts with how you prepare to cut it out.

Right side, wrong side

Your fabric has a right and a wrong side. If there is a printed pattern, this will be on the right side. If your fabric is a solid colour, you should be able to tell the right side by the selvedge (the woven edges of the fabric). From a set of rough holes on the right side. This is where the fabric was suspended in rollers during factory treatment.

Fold your fabric right sides together along the selvedges and press all over and along the fold.

Paper press

Are you working with tissue paper pattern pieces? Then turn your iron down to a cool setting and iron your pattern pieces to get rid of any creases. Creases distort shape and size, which will have an impact on fitting. This process will send static into your paper pieces from ions in the iron, but don't worry – this static soon disappears.

ANOTHER SEWING SPACE THAT YOU CAN
FILL WITH USEFUL TOOLS.
LOOK OUT FOR:

- A pressing ham - for pressing fabric that will lay over curves like shoulders or breasts.
- A pressing cloth - to avoid shiny press marks or avoid delicate fabrics from melting.
- Sleeve board - when you need to get into the seams of smaller items such as sleeves or collars.
- Wooden clapper - a game changer for pressing seams flat. These hold the steam into your fabric after pressing.

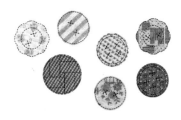

Your pressing station

Once pressed, lay your fabric out on a clean floor or table. You'll likely need to roll one end of your fabric up when you start.

- If you're working with a print that needs careful print matching, it may be worth cutting out in a single layer and flipping pattern pieces.

- Working with slippery fabrics? Then, pin the selvedges together to prevent the fabric from moving about.

- Silk is divine, but its floaty nature makes it difficult to cut out accurately. Pin silk to a sheet of paper and cut through all layers. This makes such a difference.

WHAT IS PATTERN MATCHING?

This is a technique to make sure that a repeating pattern lines up properly across seams when sewing, or to ensure that you don't end up with an unfortunate pattern over key parts of your body (think pineapples over your groin or breasts!). Tips include cutting in a single layer so that you can accurately match up each pattern piece to an identical section of the pattern, buying extra fabric to accommodate pattern matching and to match the most obvious seams first. Of course, if you buy a non-directional print (one that goes up, down and across your fabric) you won't have to worry about pattern matching at all!

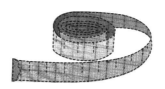

Laying out the pattern pieces

Every sewing pattern has a diagram where they show you the recommended placement of pattern pieces. Honestly, I hardly ever follow this. I lay my large pattern pieces out as close together as possible across the fabric, ensuring that they face the same way if I'm working with an obvious nap. Then I arrange the smaller pattern pieces in the gaps left.

The pattern pieces have arrows that indicate how they should be placed across the fabric's grain. This is particularly important for pieces cut on the bias.

Some pattern pieces indicate that they need to be cut on the fold. The symbol for this is a long line along one side of the pattern piece, with little arrows pointing towards the paper edge.

WHAT IS FABRIC GRAIN?

This is the warp and weft of the fabric from how the threads are woven. The warp is lengthwise grain and the weft is crosswise grain. Bias is the 45-degree angle between these threads.

It is important to make sure that fabric is laid out flat and accurately and that your pattern pieces are pinned according to the grain - so that arrows follow either the warp or the weft.

If you don't pin accurately, fabric can twist and distort the final make. Plus, it's fun measuring up the little arrows with a tape measure leading out towards the selvedge!

Attaching pattern pieces

There are a number of simple methods you can use:

- Pins
- Pattern weights

- Tins from the kitchen cupboard

- Dogs, small children or hamsters (this one's a lie)

Alternatively, you can trace pattern pieces onto your fabric using a tracing wheel and carbon paper.

Cutting out

Using either scissors or a rotary cutter, cut out each pattern piece. Make sure you cut through all layers of fabric. If your scissors are struggling with the fabric composition, switch to a different set of blades.

Make sure you snip your notches. Notches are small triangles printed on the edge of pattern pieces. These are key for lining up seams. I promise that for such small triangles, they make a big difference. Use them!

That's it. Your pattern pieces are all cut out and now you are ready to SEW!

BE KIND TO YOUR FABRIC

A final note on fabric. Be kind to it. Once you've finished your sewing project, there's lots you can do to ensure that it lives as long as it deserves to.

- Machine wash on a gentle 30-degree wash.

- Hand wash delicates with a gentle detergent.

- Air dry items on a washing line or clothes horse.

- Choose the iron setting that best suits your fabric.

- Consider using a press cloth when ironing – and *do* iron that dress you slaved over when it comes off the line.

- When putting away in drawers, make sure to use moth balls or even acid-free paper.

- Keep out of daylight when not wearing – don't let those colours fade.

- Make repairs as soon as damage appears – don't put it off.

- Consider repurposing fabric from a make you no longer wear (you can save buttons from old clothes, too).

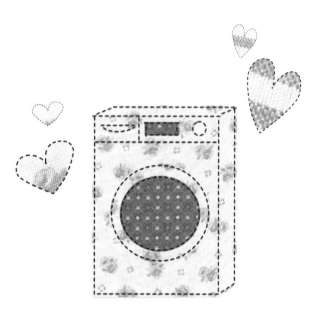

CHAPTER 6

PASSION

'Do it with passion, or not at all.'
Source unknown

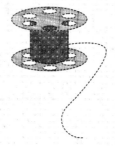

The passion creeps up on you. You dip your toe, borrow a sewing machine, make something cute. Nothing to see here, you tell yourself. It's a hobby. A nice, gentle hobby...

Next thing you know, you're sewing in your dreams, buying fabric on your lunch hour, turning down party invitations. You're addicted to sewing.

Fortunately, it's relatively harmless to indulge this passion, and you're not alone. More than 1 million people have converted to the power of a needle and thread in the past three years. That's a lot of passion.

Feeling sexy

Love your sewing machine

Sewing in books and movies

Use your sewing to change the world

Essential sewing machine accessories

Careers in sewing

For the love of sewing

You will learn:

To take care of your sewing machine
Essential sewing machine needles
Top five sewing machine feet
Other sewing machine accessories

FEELING SEXY

'To be well dressed is a little like being in love.'
Oleg Cassini

The very act of sewing involves opening up your mind and heart. The first time you consider a sewing pattern, you're inviting your imagination to see beyond the envelope illustration and envisage how this piece of clothing might look on you – or how you might look in it.

You experiment with looks you'd never normally try on in a high-street changing room – all behind closed doors as you play with fabric and thread. This can lead you down all sorts of exciting paths.

Over the years, you may have convinced yourself that you can only wear a certain type of outfit – 'I don't suit dresses' or 'I can't wear that hem length'. But once you start sewing, you find yourself exploring ideas you'd never considered before and this can lead to an explosion of sexual confidence. 'Hey, I look great in this! I feel sexy.'

Sewing can be wonderfully liberating.

Underpinnings

When was the last time you took a long, hard look at your underwear drawer? This is one of the unexpected benefits of sewing – you quickly learn the importance of decent underwear. Well-fitting undergarments are the best friends of a home-sewn outfit.

Once you start to explore the myriad options around your base layers you'll discover a whole new world of adventure. You could even sew your own...

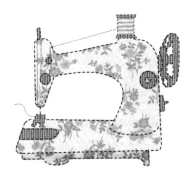

UNDERWEAR RESOURCES FOR SEWISTS

- **What Katy Did**: From satin bullet bras to lined stockings, this is the vintage lover's best friend when it comes to 1950s lingerie. Visit their website and swoon.

- **Red Fern Lingerie**: These specialize in underwear for 'sexy survivors', allowing women who have experienced breast cancer to re-engage with their femininity.

- **Madalynne Intimates**: If you want to sew your own DIY lingerie, this supplier provides kits and workshops for you to sew your own in the most gorgeous laces and satins.

- **Rigby & Peller**: Bra maker to the queen, no less! The highly trained staff at Rigby & Peller treat you to a bespoke fitting that promises to radically overhaul your idea of what bra you need. The lingerie is not cheap, but once you try them you'll never look back.

- **Translingerie**: This is an online business that caters to the transgender community.

Celebrate shape

Adolescence is the time our bodies change and we learn to clothe the shape we become. It's exciting and we experiment.

As we get older, we may convince ourselves that certain rules apply – that we can no longer wear skirts above the knee, or that we should only be seen in certain colours. The danger is we lose our experimental streak at just the time in life where we should have most confidence and other people judge us less. But sewing is your opportunity to push the boundaries. Experiment again!

Pin the hem up and see how it feels. Not so bad, huh? No one died from seeing those knees! Flirt with a recklessly plunging neckline. Test it out with a wearable toile (a practice make). Like how it looks? Go ahead, sew it up. Your décolletage is too pretty to hide.

Maybe you think your bum is too big for jeans. Well, guess what? You can sew your own jeans to accommodate your toosh and maybe you'll draw some admiring glances – of yourself in your mirror. I mean, it's not about pleasing other people, right?

And so it goes on. As you learn to sew, you learn to fit and flatter to your own body – and well-fitting clothes give you the confidence to experiment more. You'll feel a frisson of excitement and your sexuality is unleashed.

Your confidence is growing, and there's nothing more sexy than that.

Your sexy

Sexy doesn't have to be obvious. We all have complex and individual sexual identities and preferences. The great thing about sewing is that you can sew to your own sense of sexy. You might like:

- A New Look pegged skirts from the 1950s
- A dress full of flounces and petticoats
- Wearing gender fluid clothes

- Fabrics – do you like leather, chiffon or velvet?

- Secrets – no one else but you knows that your dress is lined in pure silk. Sexy, huh?

- Colour – do jewel tones do it for you, or do you prefer the romantic passion of a softer palette?

Exploring your sexuality through your clothes doesn't need to be a big, public statement. It can be very, very private.

LOVE YOUR
SEWING MACHINE

*'A sewing machine must be carefully used
if it is to give good service.'*
Remy Nicholson, *A Textbook Of Dressmaking*, 1936

If you're passionate about sewing, you need to pour love over the most important motor in your life - your sewing machine.

But if you're anything like me, you'll probably look at your sewing machine manual a couple of times when you buy the machine and then toss it into a drawer and forget about it. You take your loved one for granted. But sewing machines are like lovers - they demand attention.

Keep this book next to your machine for inspiration and flag this page for those times when you need to remind yourself how to persuade your sewing machine to purr like a kitten.

Clean after every project

Okay, even if it's not after every project, can you at least promise me you'll clean your machine when it becomes visibly dusty? Drape a dust cover over your machine when you're not using it. This doesn't need to be anything fancy; I use an offcut of old fabric. Store it away from windows or anywhere that attracts dust.

Every now and then, remove the throat plate and take a soft brush to remove dust and fluff from around the working parts of the machine.

Oil moving parts

Some machines are self-lubricating and don't need to be oiled. Check your manual. (You know, that one you threw into the back of a drawer.) If your machine does need oiling, it should have come with a small pipette of oil. Use it on the moving parts, following directions from – you guessed it – the manual.

I don't think I oiled my machine once in the first year of owning it. When I did, it was a revelation. It ran as smoothly as melted chocolate.

Top Tip: After oiling your machine, sew a scrap of fabric to clean any residual oil from moving parts before you run the risk of an oil stain on your WiP.

NEEDLE GUIDE

- **Needle size**: These vary from a 60/8 for fine fabrics, 80/12 for medium-weight fabrics and 110/18 for heavyweight fabrics. Honestly, I still don't understand these sizes! If you're as flummoxed as me, just buy a pack of assorted size needles and judge by eye. The finest needles for the finest fabrics – it's not rocket science!
- **Universal needle**: With a slightly rounded needle tip, this does what it says on the tin. You can use this needle on most projects.
- **Ballpoint or jersey needle**: This has a rounded tip, ideal for slipping between threads on jersey fabric.

- **Stretch needle**: A different beast to the ballpoint needle, the eye has a special 'scarf' allowing the needle to deal with super-stretchy and slippery fabrics such as Lycra without skipping stitches.
- **Topstitching needle**: If you want to use specialist topstitching polyester thread, you'll need a size 100 needle with an extra-large eye to accommodate the thicker thread.
- **Denim needle**: Dreaming of sewing your perfect pair of jeans? Then you'll need a denim needle - extra pointy.
- **Microtex needle**: These are my secret weapons for sewing fine fabrics. They save me so many headaches!

Change your needle

Some people change their sewing machine needle after every project. I can't claim to do that religiously, but I do always make sure I've safely got rid of an old needle so that a) I don't use it again and b) my dog doesn't eat it.

It is worth changing a needle regularly and according to the project. Blunt or bent needles catch fabric and spoil your sewing.

A professional service

Now, admittedly, it took me eight years of sewing to take my machine for its first service, but do as I say and not as I do! There are still high-street sewing machine specialists who will service your machine for you. Ask friends or online for personal recommendations. A service typically costs in the region of £80.

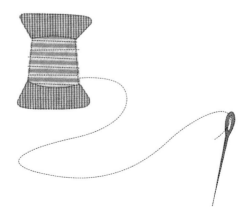

SEWING IN BOOKS
AND MOVIES

If you want to indulge your love of sewing while not actually sewing, here's a rundown of what you should read or watch.

Books

The Pink Suit, **Nicole Mary Kelly**: A fictionalized account following the dressmaker of Jackie Kennedy's infamous pink suit, worn the day her husband was assassinated.

Little House On The Prairie **series, Laura Ingalls Wilder**: If you've ever read these books, you'll remember how big an event it was to buy fabric for clothes, and then to watch Laura's mother sew for all her family.

I Capture The Castle, **Dodie Smith**: Not a big scene, but there's some brilliant dyeing of fabric and making of costumes. Regardless, this classic novel should sit beside every bedside table.

***The Button Box*, Lynn Knight**: Lynn uses an inherited box of buttons to explore her family and social history in Derbyshire. A charming journey through the decades, via the clothes – and buttons – people wore.

Movies

The Phantom Thread: A fairytale of sewing, this superb evocation of a 1950s London couturier, Reynolds Woodcock, follows Woodcock and his muse on a dark and obsessive journey. The details are gorgeous, but the show is stolen by Woodcock's sister. Perfect for a rainy afternoon of hand sewing on the sofa.

Dior And I: A fascinating 2014 documentary that follows Raf Simon as he begins work at the House of Dior. There is plenty of detail, including interviews with the *petites mains* who work there, seeing through designers' visions.

The Devil Wears Prada: Not dressmaking exactly,

but a humorous look behind the scenes of a fashion magazine, with a stand-out speech from Meryl Streep in her role as Miranda on the influence of colour in fashion. Lots of fun and a film that's become a modern classic.

The Dressmaker: Based on the novel by the same name, in this movie Kate Winslet plays, you guessed it, a dressmaker. Set in the Australian outback, we see lots of glimpses of mid twentieth-century fashion.

The Putter, **Shaun Bloodworth**: A short YouTube film about Sheffield firm Ernest Wright & Son, maker of handmade scissors.

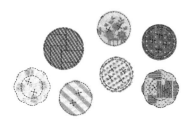

USE YOUR SEWING TO CHANGE THE WORLD

Whatever topic you feel most passionate about, sewing can help you make change. Pick a project and then think about how your sewing can help. Below are some examples of people who have used their skills powerfully for the causes they believe in.

How to be a craftivist

Award-winning campaigner Sarah Corbett grew up in a family of activists but found that conflict made her unhappy. She wanted to find a form of peaceful protest that would build bridges and turned to her embroidery hobby to launch craft campaigns and gentle protests under the umbrella of the Craftivist Collective.

Mastectomy machinists

This is a Facebook group of machine sewists who

make free drain bags and mastectomy pillows for women going through breast cancer treatment.

The Made Up Initiative

I used my blog to host a sewalong that raised over £3000 for the National Literacy Trust, a cause close to my heart. All you need to organize a similar fundraiser is a bunch of friends, a deadline and a Justgiving page. Go for it!

Slow fashion movement

You don't need to use your sewing to make a big public statement about what you believe in. Use your sewing powers to effect change in your own life. If fast fashion offends you, embrace the slow fashion movement by making your own clothes at a pace that allows you to appreciate every step of the process.

Ethical sourcing

If you're concerned about where that cheap bolt of fabric came from, there are lots of opportunities to buy organic or ethical fabric online or in shops. It might take a little extra time and thought to track these fabrics down, but your conscience will be satisfied.

Protest marches

Over recent years, these seem to have become the platform for all sorts of creativity, from posters to costumes. If you're joining a march, why don't you see what you can sew? A handmade outfit is sure to draw attention to your cause.

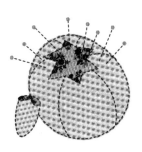

SEWING MACHINE ACCESSORIES

Is there any such thing as an essential accessory? When it comes to sewing – yes! You can never have too much of the *stuff*. It's like any hobby; half the fun is in the gathering of equipment.

I'm joking, but only partly. When it comes to your sewing machine, you'll discover there's a whole array of extra equipment you can buy. But which are the ones that count?

Five essential feet

I've bought them, I've used them, I've left them to gather dust. Which are the five sewing machine feet that work?

Standard Foot: This is what your machine comes with and is a good, all-purpose foot. Nothing to see here; move along.

Zipper Foot: This is a narrow foot that can be used to stitch closely to a zip or any other area of sewing where you need to get up close and personal.

Invisible Zipper Foot: Some people claim they can insert a perfectly invisible zip with nothing more than a standard sewing machine foot. I don't believe them. When I bought my invisible zip foot, it escalated my sewing overnight. Just buy one.

Walking Foot: Oh, how I love my walking foot! I use this more often than the standard foot. A standard sewing machine foot relies on the feed dogs' grip on the bottom layer of fabric. This means that the two layers of fabric can end up travelling through the machine at a different pace, which interferes with the accuracy of your sewing. A walking foot has two sets of grips to feed both layers of fabric through the sewing machine evenly. If you use a walking foot, you'll never again have to worry about layers of fabric shifting in the sewing machine. This can make a big difference to seam intersections and other details when you're sewing with bulky fabrics.

Buttonhole Foot: If you're going to make anything with buttonholes, unless you want to hand stitch them, you'll need a machine that can sew button-holes and you'll need a buttonhole foot. Machines either sew buttonholes automatically or as a four-step buttonhole. Either way, with a button-hole foot, you're opening yourself up to myriad new sewing opportunities. Without one, you'll need to carefully scour patterns to ensure that they don't use buttonholes.

Five other essentials

Spare Bobbins: The bobbin is a small reel that you thread, to sit beneath the presser foot and feed thread up through the feed plate. Most machines come with a few, but I find it really useful to buy spares. If your machine takes steel bobbins, these are the best. Otherwise, plastic bobbins will do. Pre-thread them in a variety of colours so that you always have a bobbin of the right thread to hand.

A Daylight Lamp: I keep one of these next to my sewing machine. On those dark, winter nights you'll need the extra light.

A Wastepaper Basket: Or you can tape a paper bag to the side of the table. Whichever, you'll need a repository close by for all those threads and fabric scraps. They build up fast, so unless you want your sewing space to look like a bird's nest, have a bin close to hand.

A Mirror: I hang a mirror on the wall above my sewing machine. It's so useful for a quick check of how something looks against my body and saves me rushing upstairs to change for the hundredth time.

Computer Cleaning Kit: Raid your office for one of these. They hold all you need to clean your sewing machine, too - soft brushes, cleaning fluid, a blower, soft duster. Job done!

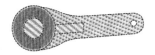

CAREERS IN SEWING

'I get so much joy seeing what my customers make. Every day is different. Some days I spend hours with suppliers choosing new stock, other days I can spend the day packing, and then there are the days that involve accounting and website admin. Starting Sew Me Sunshine took a long time to plan and a big investment, but it was definitely worth it. I am excited to see where the business will go in the years to come.'

Harriet Cleary, owner of online fabric shop,
Sew Me Sunshine

You may decide that you love sewing so much that you want to turn it into your career. After all, so many people today pursue multiple careers, pivot their career or pursue the entrepreneurial dream. Could you be a Sewing Start-up, too?

There are lots of options, but it's wise to pursue your dreams with wide-open eyes. Here are a few considerations before you march into your boss's office to hand in your notice.

Hobby or job?

When you start sewing it's your way of relaxing. If you were sewing five days a week, do you think it would still help you relax, or would you learn to hate your seam ripper? Turning your hobby into your job can drain all the joy from it.

Do you have savings?

The rule of thumb is that you should have at least six months' salary saved up before you take the leap into a new freelance lifestyle. For people living in expensive cities this can be close to impossible, but you should aim to have some financial cushion.

Business plan?

Starting a new working life takes research and planning over pipe dreams. If you're setting up on your own, you should write a business plan and a projected first year's cash flow. If you don't know how to do either of these, learn. There are loads of resources out there, from the British Library IP Centre to Enterprise Nation, and great conferences such as Blogtacular.

Part time?

This is an excellent way of testing the water. You don't have to walk away from your current job straight away. You could try some part-time work on evenings or weekends to test your level of commitment. If you don't like the new way of working, you still have the security of your original salary.

Support network?

Changing career direction can be extremely taxing. Do you have friends and family close by to support you? Someone to cook the evening meal when you're too tired? A pet to cuddle you at the end of the day? Support systems matter, so make sure yours is in place.

Brainstorm!

This is the fun bit – gather some friends and brainstorm ideas for what your new way of working could be. No idea is wrong, just throw them out there and then you can fine tune.

Does it need to be now?

Are you the type of person who has a five-year plan? (I'm totally not, by the way!) If you are, you could work your new career direction into your plan. You don't need to march into the office and hand in your notice tomorrow. A word to the wise, though: once you've made a firm decision about your life direction, it's very hard to keep turning up to the current office.

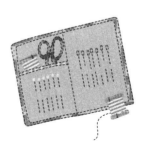

PODCASTS FOR SEWING ENTREPRENEURS

- **The Stitcher's Brew**: Gabby and Megan often interview sewing business leaders about how they went about building a new enterprise from scratch. Listen and learn.

- **In Good Company**: Otegha Uwagba is the author of bestselling *The Little Black Book* and interviews inspirational women who have forged successful new entrepreneurial paths for themselves. Full of sound and sensible advice.

- **While She Naps**: Abby Glassenberg has built herself a reputation as a reliable journalist in the crafting sphere. Alongside her careful research, she often asks the questions no one else will. Great for an accurate, contemporary view of the crafting industry.

- **Blogtacular**: With a focus on online creative endeavour, these podcasts regularly interview crafters full of inspiration and stories about both failures and successes.

Career Options

There are loads of sewing careers out there – you just need to choose the right one for you. You may discover that you end up with a portfolio career, juggling several of these options.

Teaching Sewing: Most often, this takes place in sewing studios. This is a good option if you need mentoring in the early days of your teaching career. If you choose to teach independently, make sure you have public liability insurance and that you are fully prepared. How will you make up the shortfall if customers cancel bookings?

Online Fabric Shop: Several of these have launched over recent years. You'll need great web-building abilities (or to know a reliable IT whizz), suppliers, a cash float and somewhere to store stock.

Sewing Pattern Designer: If you have training in pattern cutting, you could release your own sewing patterns. It might be sensible to do this digitally in the first instance, with PDF downloads to test the market. You'll need a certain amount of audience to ensure people know your patterns exist and that there's an appetite to buy them. I'd suggest you also need a strong sense of your aesthetic and what your USP is in a crowded marketplace.

Sewing Journalism Or Writing: See these as supplementary strands to your career, and not as a main breadwinner. Journalism and writing are great marketing tools to raise your profile and, in the long term, can bring in royalty income if you engage with traditional book publishing, but these streets are largely not paved with gold!

Self Publishing: This is an option, and it can be a profitable one, but key to any self-publishing project is accurate costing and then knowing how to reach your audience. Anyone can write a book, but how do you get people to know about it? If you're going down this route, you should take the marketing and publicity as seriously as you do the writing – and this can become more than a full-time job.

Sponsorship: If your social media channel of choice gets a large enough audience, you may be able to charge for advertising, either with sponsored blog buttons or affiliate marketing. Transparency is key and, again, I would advise seeing this as an income thread but not as your main source of money.

CAN YOU AFFORD IT?

This is my most important question to you. Will you be able to pay the bills each month if you pursue your dream? Sit down and do some sums before you even start planning an escape from the rat race.

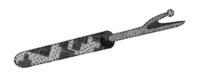

FOR THE LOVE OF SEWING

'Hello my darling, I got the sweetest letter
today from the sweetest little angel on
earth. You do write wonderful letters,
sweetheart and they tell me just what
I want to hear, that you love me.
I am so very fortunate to have you love
me, little one. I don't know what I did
to deserve this, such wonderful love,
but I don't question it.
Your loving husband — Forever, Walter'
Sgt. First Class Walter Smith, 1963

This love note was found hidden inside a vintage sewing machine. When was the last time you looked inside yours?

Sewing can be the most romantic of pastimes and there are some gorgeous stories about how people share their love and passion through sewing.

Consider these next time you're in a romantic mood.

Love notes

Swoon! Truly, the vintage buyer's dream – to find a sewing pattern that contains a long-forgotten love letter. Or maybe you'd prefer to leave a note for the sewist in your life? Just slip it into that little paper envelope and wait to see how long it takes your loved one to find it.

Beyond romance

'Here's a pillowcase, stitched in blue, just a reminder that I love you.'
(Embroidered into a pillowcase for blog reader Lin, by her mother.)

Love notes can be more than romantic – they can be for your children or family members. Here's an example of a note left for a teenage child going off to college. Wouldn't a secret message like this be the best comfort for a homesick student?

Hidden messages

You can sew hidden messages in the seam allowances, beneath collars or into the guts of a finished make. What message would you leave for only your loved one to know about?

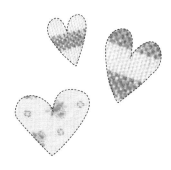

CHAPTER 7

HIGHS
AND LOWS

*'I haven't failed, I've just found 10,000
ways that don't work'*
Thomas Edison

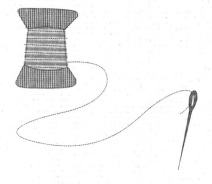

I thought I'd finished writing this book, but I hadn't. After I attended a sewing retreat along with 200 other enthusiasts I realized I'd failed to cover every range of sewing emotions.

At that retreat, I burnt my fabric, inserted a sleeve wrong and swore more times than was sociable. I was frustrated with my own sewing. I might even have thrown the fabric on the floor.

I had a thunderbolt of clarity. *The Little Book Of Sewing* would only be half a book if I didn't cover the more challenging emotions around sewing. So, let's see what can go wrong and how we feel about it.

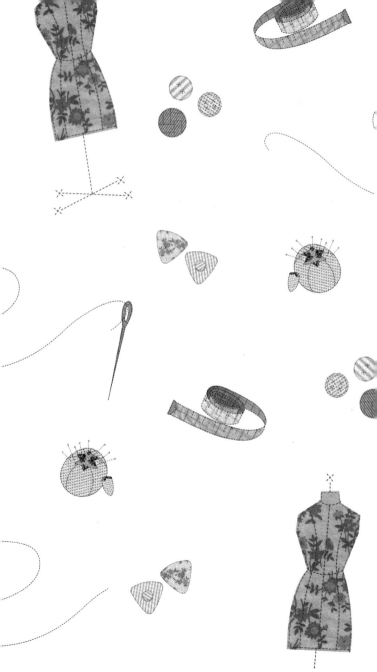

Ten most common sewing mistakes

How to handle sewing frustration

Advice you can afford to ignore

What to do with failed projects

Remember...

You will learn:

How to insert a sleeve

Hand stitching secrets

How to place pocket bags

To avoid gaping buttons

TEN MOST COMMON
SEWING MISTAKES

Hey, look – I can't claim to have done years of rigorous research under controlled conditions. These are the mistakes that I've either made myself or observed in others. Mistakes happen a lot – that's why the seam ripper was invented. Welcome to a rundown of the sewing mistakes you're likely to make in front of the sewing machine at some point in your sewing career. Don't say I didn't warn you!

1) Scorching fabric

A decent iron is one of your best sewing tools. Ask me how I know. I've had more fabric be burnt with a too-hot iron than I care to think about. I've also suffered the consequences of an iron spitting hard-water residue. Believe me, it all starts (and sometimes ends) at the ironing board.

Top Tip: Go middle-of-the-range when buying an iron. You don't need to spend big on one of those super-duper gravity feeds thingummybobs. Nor should you buy the cheapest iron you can find secondhand on an internet auction site. Spend a little more than you might normally, and you'll save yourself a whole lot of headache. Believe me, I speak from experience.

2) Using a blunt needle

Sometimes the biggest problems can come from the tiniest sources. When was the last time you changed the needle in your machine? Why do you keep stabbing that blunt pin back into your pincushion?

Top Tip: It's not rocket science, people. Change the needle in your machine with every project. When you notice that a pin is blunt, toss it. It takes 30 seconds of your life, possibly less.

3) Forcing a machine

Ever had that knot of thread at the start of a row of stitching? Buttonholes giving you grief? Tension all wrong? It's easy to keep on sewing despite the (often noisy) evidence that your machine just isn't happy. And then you wonder why your seam line puckers.

Top Tip: Don't be stubborn. Take a deep breath and take the thread out of your machine. The spool and the bobbin both. Yes, both! Rethread the whole machine from scratch. Nine times out of ten, this solves whatever the problem was.

4) Fitting issues

Fit is arguably the most challenging part of sewing. Our bodies are unique. The way that shoulders, chest, waist and hips translate to a sewing pattern can feel overwhelming when you're trying to sew an outfit that fits.

Top Tip: If you're unsure of fit, sew a toile (muslin) first. A toile is a test make that allows you to tweak before cutting into your prized fashion fabric. Choose a cheap fabric in a similar weight and drape to the fabric you've chosen for your final make. Sew it in long, tacking stitches that allow you to rip out seams and adjust quickly.

5) Wrong sleeve, wrong armhole

I do this. All. The. Time. And guys, sleeves are hard to sew in! I always tack first and I'm always glad I did. Still, I make this mistake way too often.

Top Tip: Do transfer the sleeve head notches from pattern piece to cut-out fabric. Notice how one side of the sleeve head has one notch and the other has two notches? One notch means the sleeve should go to the front of your arm, and two notches indicate the back pattern piece. There's more room in the back section of the sleeve head to accommodate your shoulder joint and movement, so don't ignore these notches!

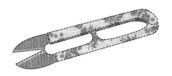

6) Tight hand stitching

Sometimes your own little couture touch can be a hand-sewn hem, working on the wrong side of the fabric so that your stitches are invisible on the right side. When I started sewing, I believed that tight stitches were the best route to exemplary sewing. I was wrong in my belief. All they do is bunch the fabric up and make the stitching even more obvious.

Top Tip: Channel your inner yogi and take a relaxed approach to hand stitches when hemming a skirt or trousers. My favourite hand stitch for hemming is the catch stitch, sewn in loose Vs.

7) Sewing under the influence

A debatable topic! Do you sew with a glass of wine next to your machine? Some people love this as part of the winding-down process; others can't concentrate once a sip of wine has passed their lips. Know your limits!

Top Tip: If a misted glass of something cold and

dry is your acknowledged reward system, keep it for the end of your sewing session.

8) Pocket bags too low

Pockets are a feminist issue – discuss! If a sewing pattern doesn't come with pockets, it's often simple enough to insert them in the side seams. You can use a pocket bag pattern piece from another project – but make sure you don't sew them too low into the seam line. Remember that the bottom, not the top, of your pocket bag is where your hand will sit.

Top Tip: Pin the pocket bag pattern piece to your skirt or trouser side seam and then measure the placement against where your hand naturally falls by your side. Your fist should sit in the base of the pocket bag.

9) Button placement

If you're sewing a buttoned shirt dress or shirt, the placement of buttons is crucial to gapes around your boobage. It's a pain to have spent hours on a pattern, only to discover that it gapes across your bra.

Top Tip: I often ignore button placing suggestions that come with a pattern. Try on your make and see where the bodice lies across your chest. Place a button at the fullest part to avoid any unseemly gapes.

10) Wonky topstitching

Topstitching is a row of stitching on the right side of the garment, used as a decorative feature. Think about the golden topstitching you see on indigo jeans. There's nothing more eye-catching than a row of topstitching that's as wobbly as an ocean wave! It's easy to be seduced by topstitching; less easy to execute it accurately. I'd suggest being cautious around contrast topstitching unless you're confident of accuracy.

Top Tip: For accuracy, you don't necessarily need to invest in specialist sewing machine feet. Eyeball a section of your sewing machine foot that runs parallel to the seam line you are topstitching and keep that section accurately running along your seam line as you stitch.

HOW TO HANDLE SEWING FRUSTRATION

'A wonky hem isn't because of lack of skill or knowledge. It's about not being patient enough to do it un-wonky.'
Blog reader, Stina P

It takes 10,000 hours to become really good at something. That's 9,999 hours of making mistakes. Tell me about it!

How do you handle the anger and tears that can accompany sewing? When you're just not feeling it and want to sell your machine to the nearest buyer?

Go for a walk

This is pretty much my answer to every problem in life, but half an hour away from your machine can do you the world of good. Fresh air, thinking time, peace and quiet. Whenever I go for a walk, I always return home struggling to remember what had made me so angry.

Know when to schedule

Sewists have a canny knack of giving themselves unrealistic deadlines. Wedding tomorrow? I'll start making a dress! Yeah, that's largely going to end up being one knotty pit of misery. If I have a big sewing project, I always try to schedule. Then I build in wasted time, as I would with any professional project. Then I add an extra week. On top of that, I try to sew in chunks of time, understanding when my brain is too tired to continue.

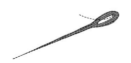

Accept imperfection

The likelihood of you sewing the perfectly perfect item of clothing is close to nil. Why do we find vintage handmade garments so charming? Because we can see the hand stitches and spot the imperfections. Even in the couture garments that I've seen up close, you can often see when a row of stitches are not all religiously consistent. Mergh. It's no biggie. Just be the best that you can be.

Find inspiration elsewhere

A bad day sewing? Pack up the machine and do something else instead. You could build a Pinterest mood board, engage with other sewists on Instagram, snoop the construction of clothes in high-street stores.

Compare to other hobbies

With running, the more hours you put in the better you get. Why does it have to be any different with sewing? Just accept that it will take a certain number of hours to get to where you want to be – and then enjoy the journey. Learning new skills is fun!

Take a class

If you feel as though you've hit a brick wall in terms of what you can teach yourself, consider taking a class. Not only will you learn great skills and tips from your teacher, who will be able to help you fit, but you'll make some great new sewing pals. Win, win!

Invest in high-end fabric

This is a clever way of tricking your brain into taking your sewing more seriously. If you spend some precious disposable income on gorgeous fabric, you might force yourself to slow down and take sewing seriously.

Keep yourself happy

It's easy to see a sewing pattern made up by someone else and fall in love. You buy the pattern, sew your own version and... oh, disappointment. Remember that, with time, you'll learn to judge what suits your body and lifestyle. Sewing is not an Instagram FOMO moment – it's what you're doing to keep yourself happy.

Remember – it's just fabric. No one died.

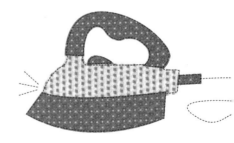

ADVICE YOU CAN AFFORD TO IGNORE

There's a lot of advice on the Internet, aimed at new sewists. Everyone's an expert – and how do you unpick sound advice from pearl-clutching hysteria? I'm throwing my hat into the ring to suggest that there are some pieces of advice you can afford to ignore. May the Gods Of Sewing smite me down! There are no rules. Just do what works for you.

Never sew over pins

There are dangers here and I'm not going to advocate merrily speed sewing over bunches of pins. A machine can be damaged or, worse, a pin breaks and flies into your eye. Be careful: slow the machine right down and remove each pin just before your machine needle sews over it. But you don't always need to tack first.

Tailor's chalk

Tailor's chalk – half the stuff I buy never works. And really, can't you mark fabric with anything? Lead pencil, Sharpie, biro, felt tip, crayon – if it makes a mark and you're working within a seam allowance, you can use anything! If you're marking fabric in areas of the finished make, do be sure it shall wash out first. Otherwise, draw away!

Press immediately

Sure, the iron is a sewist's best friend. But do you need to hop over to the ironing board after every seam has been sewn? Not necessarily. You can batch iron a bunch of work, waiting until you've finished a few sewing steps. Or you can finger press seams in certain fabrics, simply using the pressure and heat of your fingertips. It really works!

Use a press cloth

A press cloth protects delicate fabrics from the

sheen that an iron's plate can leave behind. Mostly, I use a silk organza press cloth because its diaphanous weave allows me to see my work through the cloth and silk stands up to a high heat. If I don't happen to have a press cloth to hand? I use a clean tea towel! We don't always need to overthink our equipment.

Buy the best

Sure, on occasion. But you don't always need to spend mega bucks on fabric. Visit your local market, car boot sale or charity shop. There's always cheap fabric to practise on or even create stunning final pieces from.

WHAT TO DO WITH FAILED PROJECTS

Sometimes we make something we never wear. Either it doesn't fit properly or we just don't like it. But, wait! Don't toss that outfit in the bin. You spent hours sewing it and that would be a waste of good fabric.

Gift it to someone else

My younger sister has a slimmer figure than me, so if I sew something too small it goes to the pile of clothes I take to her whenever I visit. Honestly, I never really know if she wears these items or if they go straight to the charity shop. I don't really care – it makes me feel better about wasted sewing time.

Take it to the charity shop

Plenty of sewists derive real pleasure from spotting their handmade items proudly displayed in the window of a charity shop – and then quickly bought. Don't forget that the dress you detest, someone else might love. Think of the extra thrill the new owner will receive when he or she realizes their new purchase is hand made.

Refashion it

If there's enough fabric in the finished make, you may be able to rescue sections to turn into a different item. Swishy dresses and skirts are your friend. Or you could add elements to the project to transform it into something else entirely. There's a wealth of refashioning knowledge on the Internet.

Rename it as a toile!

A less than successful make can be your practice run. Just tell people you were testing the make before cutting into your final version. Take note of adjustments and lessons learned and start again. Hey, you were just practising!

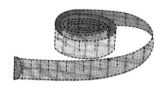

REMEMBER

You are awesome and everything you've sewn and achieved is magnificent. These aren't empty words. How many people do you know who can create a 3-D object to place around their body? Your ability with a needle and thread makes you unique. It also means you have the skills to clothe yourself and your loved ones when that zombie apocalypse happens. Good times!

There is no failure in sewing, only learning, community, creative inspiration and happiness. Okay, maybe sometimes a bit of swearing. But mainly happiness.

Thank you so much for reading *The Little Book of Sewing* and going on this journey through the emotions that hit us all when we pick up a needle.

Now, what are you going to sew next...?

RESOURCES:

KEEP
GOING!

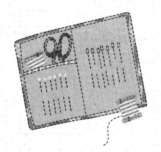

If you're inspired to do more sewing, here's a rundown of some of my favourite resources. Don't forget to share your inspired makes with new and familiar friends on social media using the hashtags #littlebookofsewing #passionintofashion.

I can't wait to see your achievements.

Online fabric shops

www.bobbinsnbuttons.co.uk

www.clothspot.co.uk

www.dittofabrics.co.uk

www.dragonflyfabrics.co.uk

www.fabricgodmother.co.uk

www.girlcharlee.co.uk

www.likesewamazing.com

www.minervacrafts.com

www.moodfabrics.com

www.aystitch.co.uk

www.thesewcialstudio.co.uk

www.sewmesunshine.co.uk

www.sewoverit.co.uk

www.stoffstil.co.uk

www.stonefabrics.co.uk

www.stonemountainfabric.com

www.thimbleandnotch.co.uk

www.thevillagehaberdashery.co.uk

For hints and tips around fabric, read the Fabric Focus series on my blog at www.didyoumakethat.com

Sewing pattern companies

The Big Four:

Butterick

McCalls

Simplicity

Vogue

My favourite indie pattern companies:

Deer & Doe

Named Clothing

Sew Over It

Tessuti

Tilly and the Buttons

True Bias

Sewing books I recommend

No Patterns Needed, Rosie Martin, Laurence King, 2016

The Reader's Digest New Complete Guide To Sewing, Reader's Digest, 2003

The Maker's Atelier, Frances Tobin, Quadrille, 2017

Love At First Stitch, Tilly Walnes, Quadrille, 2014

Stretch, Tilly Walnes, Quadrille, 2018

Breaking The Pattern: A Modern Way To Sew, Saara Huhta and Laura Huhta, Quadrille, 2018

Sewing Magazines

Burda: a German monthly magazine with reams of traceable sewing patterns.

The Maker's Atelier: a self-published quarterly magazine, beautifully produced.

Lisa Comfort: another self-published quarterly magazine from the founder of Sew Over It.

Love Sewing: monthly issues with free patterns.

Suzy: an indie magazine run by Dominque Major and Rosa Angelica.

Threads: a monthly in-depth bible.

Sewing blogs I enjoy

www.almondrock.co.uk

www. englishgirlathome.com

www.ericabunker.com

www.thefoldline.com/blog

www.oonaballoona.com

www.ooobop.com

www.sunnygalstudio.blogspot.com

www.tillyandthebuttons.com

www.whatkatiesews.net

www.whileshenaps.com

THANK YOU

To the lovely team at Head of Zeus, especially my editor, Ellen. Also, big thanks to the small but mighty team at Speckled Pen. And, of course, to the many passionate and loyal blog readers who have contributed to *Did You Make That* over the years. Some of you allowed me to share your sewing quotes in this book.

Most of all, to my family for their constant support and cheerleading.

notes

....
....
....
....
....
....
....
....
....
....
....
....
....
....
....
....
....

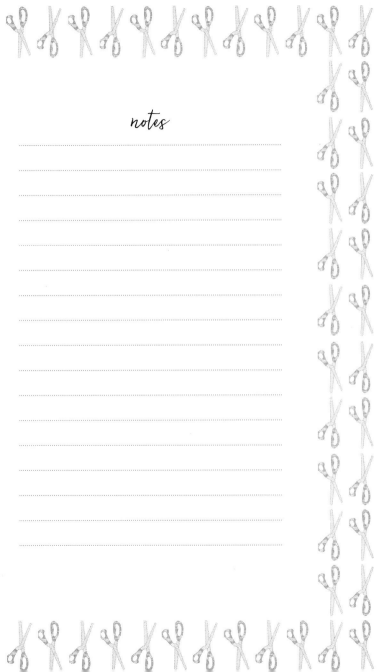

notes

···
···
···
···
···
···
···
···
···
···
···
···
···
···
···
···
···

notes

....
....
....
....
....
....
....
....
....
....
....
....
....
....
....
....
....

notes

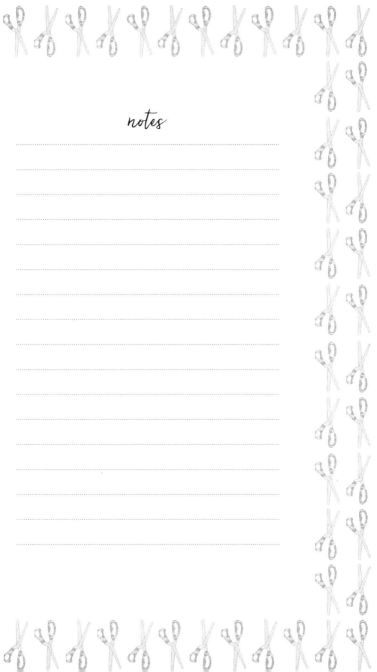

notes

notes

....

....

....

....

....

....

....

....

....

....

....

....

....

....

....

....

....

....

ABOUT THE AUTHOR

Karen Ball runs the leading sewing blog, *Did You Make That*, and has written about sewing for *The Guardian*, and for *Love Sewing*, *Sewing World* and *Sew* magazines. She is the author of over twenty books and runs the publishing consultancy, Speckled Pen. She was nominated a Rising Star by *The Bookseller* in 2017. She lives in London with her miniature schnauzer, Ella.